Study Guide to Accompany

Pillitteri's Maternal and Child Health Nursing

CARE OF THE CHILDBEARING AND CHILDREARING FAMILY

FOURTH EDITION

PREPARED BY

Joyce Young Johnson, R.N., Ph.D., C.C.R.N.

Assistant Chair
Department of Nursing
Georgia Perimeter College
Clarkston, Georgia

President and CEO
Johnson Consulting
Atlanta, Georgia

Edna Boyd-Davis, R.N., B.S.N., M.N.

Nurse Consultant
United States Army Nurse Corps
Chief Nurse
3297th USAH
Fort McPherson, Georgia

Visit the Lippincott Williams & Wilkins Website
http://www.lww.com

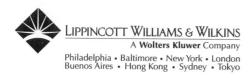
LIPPINCOTT WILLIAMS & WILKINS
A **Wolters Kluwer** Company
Philadelphia • Baltimore • New York • London
Buenos Aires • Hong Kong • Sydney • Tokyo

Ancillary Editor: Doris S. Wray
Compositor: LWW
Printer/Binder: Victor

ISBN: 0-7817-4017-7

To my husband Larry, my daughter Virginia, and my son Larry Jr. who make life worth living; and to my parents, sisters, brother, and best friends who support and nurture me and whose faith in me continues to motivate me.

Joyce Young Johnson

To my son and daughter, Jakara and Monica, of whom I am so very proud.

To the memory of my parents and brother who encouraged, loved, and nurtured me so intently.

To my brother, Roy Ishman Mitchell, who has been there for me always and has taught me the value of patience.

Edna Boyd-Davis

To our students, who are the reasons we do what we do.

Contributors

Gloria Johns, R.N., M.S.N, N.P.
Instructor, Pediatric Nursing
Department of Nursing
Georgia Perimeter College
Clarkston, Georgia

Muriel G. Mitchell, R.N., M.S.N.
Assistant Professor, Pediatric Nursing
Department of Nursing
Georgia Perimeter College
Clarkston, Georgia

Preface

The student workbook is designed to accompany the fourth edition of *Maternal and Child Health Nursing: Care of the Childbearing and Childrearing Family* by Adele Pillitteri. The workbook material directly addresses the units in the textbook and provides exercises to assist the student in learning important terms and concepts. Some anatomy, physiology, and pathophysiology concepts are addressed; however, a major focus is the role nurses play in helping the nation meet health goals by providing a quality maternal-newborn and child health nursing care. The use of the nursing process to address the physiological and psychosocial needs of the client and family in a holistic and culturally appropriate manner is addressed by the questions in this workbook.

The workbook is divided into chapters that correlate with those in the text. Each chapter includes a brief review of the chapter, along with the student learning objectives and a list of key terms for the chapter. The questions are divided into four sections. Section One addresses the use of key terms and concepts introduced in the chapters. Section Two provides completion and short answer questions. Section Three allows the student an opportunity to think critically by answering multiple choice questions with client situations or by determining the appropriateness of select nursing implementations. In addition, Section Three contains a case study with questions designed to encourage students to continue to focus on clinical application of core content. Section Four contains two parts. The first provides additional activities for inquiry (e.g., developing a teaching plan or nursing care plan or contrasting two methods of care); the second suggests activities for exploration of nursing care priorities in clinical settings and the community at large.

Questions in the workbook vary from matching and fill-in-the-blank, to true/false and multiple choice, to questions that require a longer explanation. Enough space is provided to answer most questions, but some students may find it necessary to use a separate sheet of paper to provide in-depth responses to some of the short-answer questions. Answers to objective questions are included at the back of the book.

Case studies and related questions are designed to stimulate critical thinking as well as test knowledge and principles; therefore, no answers are provided. Students can work through them on a separate sheet of paper. Instructors may also find case studies particularly useful for classroom discussion as well.

The instructor may assign an entire workbook chapter or parts of the chapter, as needed. We hope that both the text and workbook provide the student with an opportunity to fully explore and learn about the important concepts of maternal-newborn and child health nursing.

Joyce Young Johnson, Ph.D., R.N.
Edna Boyd-Davis, R.N., B.S.N., M.N.

Acknowledgments

We would like to thank Doris Wray for her support and assistance during the production of this manuscript. We would like to thank Clemmie Riggins and LaGretta Walton afor their vauluable service in the preparation of this manuscript.

Contents

UNIT V
The Nursing Role in Caring for the Family During the Postpartal Period

UNIT VI
The Nursing Role in Health Promotion for the Childrearing Family

UNIT VII
The Nursing Role in Supporting the Health of Ill Children and Their Families

UNIT VIII
The Nursing Role in Restoring and Maintaining the Health of Children and Families With Physiologic Disorders

UNIT IX

The Nursing Role in Restoring and Maintaining the Health of Children and Families With Mental Health Disorders

UNIT I

Maternal and Child Health Nursing Practice

A Framework For Maternal and Child Health Nursing

CHAPTER OVERVIEW

Chapter 1 presents an overview of maternal and child health nursing. The use of nursing process, nursing research, and nursing theory in the provision of quality care is discussed. The standards of nursing practice and the varied roles assumed by nurses in maternal and child health nursing are also explored.

LEARNING OBJECTIVES

After mastering the contents of this chapter, you should be able to:

1. Identify the goals and philosophy of maternal and child health nursing.

2. Describe the evolution, scope, and professional roles for nurses in maternal and child health nursing.

3. Define common statistical terms used in the field, such as infant and maternal mortality.

4. Discuss the implications of the common standards of maternal and child health nursing and the health goals for the nation for maternal and child health nursing practice.

5. Discuss the interplay of nursing process, evidence-based practice, and nursing theory as they relate to the future of maternal and child health nursing practice.

6. Use critical thinking to identify areas of care that could benefit from additional nursing research.

7. Integrate knowledge of trends in maternal and child health care with the nursing process to achieve an understanding of quality maternal and child health nursing care.

KEY TERMS

clinical nurse specialist
evidence-based practice
family nurse practitioner
fertility rate
maternal and child health nursing
maternal-newborn nursing
mortality
mortality rate

neonatal nurse practitioner
neonate
nurse-midwife
nursing research
pediatric nurse practitioner
puerperium
scope of practice
women's health practitioner

■ Section One:
Identification of Key Terms and Concepts

PART 1

Match the terms in Part A with a definition or related statement from Part B. Place the letter corresponding to the answer in the space provided.

PART A

1. _____ Maternal and child nursing

2. _____ Health promotion

3. _____ Nursing research

4. _____ Primary goal of maternal and child health nursing

5. _____ Health restoration

6. _____ Standards of maternal and child health nursing practice

7. _____ Puerperium

8. _____ Evidence-based practice

PART B

A. Guidelines developed by the American Nurses Association and Association of Women's Health, Obstetric, and Neonatal Nurses

B. Promptly diagnosing and treating illness using interventions that will return the client to wellness most rapidly

C. Controlled investigation of problems that has implications for nursing practice

D. Involves care of a woman before conception and through pregnancy, and care of the child prenatally, from birth and the neonatal period, and from infancy through adolescence

E. The 6-week period following childbirth; the "fourth trimester"

F. Involves the use of research as a foundation of action

G. Educating clients to be aware of good health through teaching and role modeling

H. The promotion and maintenance of optimal family health to ensure cycles of optimal childbearing and childrearing

PART 2

Match the major concept of each theory found in Part A with the theorist's name found in Part B. Place the letter corresponding to the theorist's name in the space provided. (Letters may be used only once; some letters may not be used.)

PART A

1. _____ Nursing is a process of action, reaction, interaction, and transaction.

2. _____ The role of nursing is to structure elements of the environment to give the client the best chance for recovery.

3. _____ A person comprises subsystems that must remain in balance for optimal functioning.

4. _____ Nursing is aimed at reducing stressors through primary, secondary, and tertiary prevention.

5. _____ The focus of nursing is on the individual's ability to complete self-care.

PART B

A. Dorothea Orem

B. Imogene King

C. Florence Nightingale

D. Betty Neuman

E. Sister Callistra Roy

F. Dorothy Johnson

G. Hildegard Peplau

■ Section Two: Short Answer and Completion Exercises

PART 1

Complete the following short answer exercises.

1. Discuss two of six trends in maternal and child health nursing care and the implications for nurses.

2. Explain the effect shorter hospital stays will have on patient care planning for a child during the postoperative period, particularly on patient and family teaching.

3. Discuss methods of promoting empowerment of parents and children in the health care setting.

PART 2

Complete the following fill-in-the-blank exercises.

1. The leading causes of neonatal infant mortality are _____, _____, _____, _____, and _____ _____.

2. Early hospital discharge has resulted in many women and children returning home _____ they are fully ready to _____ themselves.

3. The _____ _____ _____ is skilled in the care of the newborn, both ill and well.

4. The nurse must understand the _____ of practice, which is the range of services and care that may be provided by the nurse based on state requirements.

■ Section Three: Critical Thinking for Application of Essential Concepts

PART 1

Circle the letter corresponding to the appropriate answer.

1. Maternal mortality is defined as
   A. the number of fetal deaths occurring as a result of maternal negligence during pregnancy.
   B. the number of maternal deaths per 100,000 live births that occur as a direct result of the reproductive process.
   C. the number of pregnancies per 1,000 women that result in maternal death.
   D. the number of fetal deaths (fetus weight over 500 g) per 1,000 live births resulting in maternal death.

2. A newly admitted patient expresses a wish to continue taking the herbal medicine he brought from home to help relieve his abdominal pain. Which of the following would be an appropriate reply?
   A. "You shouldn't believe in alternative therapies; they don't work as well as modern medications."
   B. "The doctor won't like it if you take any medication other than that prescribed."
   C. "You can take the herbal medication, but only after you've taken the prescribed medications I bring to you."
   D. "We have to check the herbal treatment to be sure it doesn't interfere with prescribed medications."

3. Which of the following represents an important implication for nursing as it relates to the regionalization of pediatric care?
   A. Being away from home represents a fun adventure to children, so the nurse must ensure that the child takes health care seriously.
   B. Having the family members in a different city will allow for better bonding between the child and the hospital staff.
   C. Regionalization allows the nurse to isolate the child from parental overprotectiveness, which might slow development.
   D. The nurse has the responsibility to see that children and parents feel as welcome in the regional center as they would in a small hospital.

4. Since health care consumers are increasingly discriminating in their demands, the nurse providing maternal-child health care should do which of the following to facilitate empowerment of consumers?

   A. Allow minimal input from the client and family members into the planning of care to prevent excessive interference.

   B. Keep family members informed and help them make decisions about their child's care.

   C. Limit family visitation to prevent collaboration with the client and discovery of minor errors in care.

   D. Remind the client and family members that in the hospital setting, the nurse is in charge.

5. Which of the following is an accurate description of an expanded role for nurses in maternal-child health?

   A. Clinical nurse specialists are prepared at the baccalaureate degree level and are capable of independent care of children.

   B. If a pediatric nurse practitioner (PNP) determines that a child has a major illness, the PNP can independently prescribe appropriate medication.

   C. Nurse-midwives can assume full responsibility for the care and management of women with uncomplicated pregnancies.

   D. Pediatric nurse practitioners are registered nurses who are usually prepared at the associate degree level.

6. Which of the following is an example of the implications for nursing as related to the trends of increasing concern regarding health care costs?

   A. The average American can afford to hire a nurse practitioner instead of a physician to provide less expensive but more comprehensive family health care.

   B. Nurses must become more cost-conscious about supplies and services and help reduce cost while maintaining quality care.

   C. Health care is less expensive today since most families have begun to participate in health promotion activities using primary care nurses.

   D. Financial ability to pay for services is usually unrelated to the tendency of a woman to seek and obtain prenatal care.

PART 2: CASE STUDY

Chin Won, age 26, presents at the community health center in her last trimester of pregnancy for her initial prenatal care visit. She is found to have an elevated blood pressure and excessive swelling in her legs and feet. The fetus appears small on the sonogram.

1. What are some reasons that early prenatal care might have helped to decrease Chin Won's risk for maternal mortality and perinatal mortality?

2. What measures might the nurse take to ensure that Chin Won's care is family-centered?

3. How might cultural assessment be beneficial when planning with Chin Won for health restoration and maintenance throughout the pregnancy and puerperium?

4. How would the plan of care look if Chin Won were a single woman, a working mother, or a teen?

■ Section Four: Inquiry and Exploration

PART 1: CRITICAL INQUIRY EXERCISES

1. Write a brief statement on your opinion regarding termination of pregnancy when the woman is at risk from the pregnancy and the fetus is healthy.

2. Prepare a plan for establishing an environment in which a hospitalized child can maintain a sense of parenting and family security. Include discussions of room appearance, visiting arrangements, care schedule, and input into care activities.

PART 2: CRITICAL EXPLORATION EXERCISES

Examine the policy at a local maternal-child care facility regarding the procedure a nurse must follow if she suspects that a woman and her children are victims of an abusive male family member.

The Childbearing and Childrearing Family and Community

CHAPTER OVERVIEW

Chapter 2 provides a description of the family and how nursing is involved in family-centered care. The types of families and family tasks are described according to Duvall and Miller (1990). The importance of providing nursing care that addresses families at their level of understanding, as indicated by their stage of development, is well demonstrated. This chapter challenges the student to use the community assessment tool to assist him or her in determining the relation of the family to the community. The student is instructed to use the outcome criteria to formulate a nursing plan of care. A case study is presented to provide the student with the principles of parenting as they relate to the adopted child.

LEARNING OBJECTIVES

After mastering the contents of this chapter, you should be able to:

1. Describe family structure, function, and family roles.

2. Assess a family for structure and health.

3. Formulate nursing diagnoses related to family health.

4. Develop outcome criteria to assist a family to achieve optimal health.

5. Plan health teaching strategies, such as helping a family modify its lifestyle to accommodate an ill child.

6. Implement nursing care, such as teaching a family more effective wellness behaviors.

7. Evaluate outcome criteria for achievement and effectiveness of nursing care to be certain that goals have been achieved.

8. Identify National Health Goals related to the family and specific ways that nurses can help the nation achieve these goals.

9. Identify areas of care related to family nursing that could benefit from additional nursing research or the application of evidence-based practice.

10. Use critical thinking to analyze additional ways that nursing care can be family-centered or that client care can better include family members.

11. Integrate knowledge of family nursing with nursing process to promote quality maternal and child health nursing care.

KEY TERMS

community	family of orientation
ecomap	family of procreation
family	family theory
family nursing	genogram

■ Section One:
Identification of Key Terms and Concepts

MATCHING

Match the developmental characteristics described in Part B with one of Duvall and Miller's stages of development of the family life cycle in Part A.

PART A

1. _____ Adolescence

2. _____ Early childbearing

3. _____ Marriage

4. _____ Preschool

5. _____ Retirement

PART B

A. An important nursing role is health education concerning well-child care. The nurse should also assess the parents' ability to care for an infant with health problems.

B. Accidents involving children are a major health concern, and growth and development needs and safety considerations are increased.

C. Older family members are more likely to suffer from chronic and disabling conditions than are younger members.

D. Members of the family work to obtain a mutually satisfying marriage, relate well to their families, and plan for parenthood.

E. Accidents, homicide, and suicide are the major causes of death. The nurse has an important role in facilitating communication between family members and spends time counseling them on safety, proper care of and respect for firearms, and drug abuse.

■ Section Two:
Short Answer and Completion Exercises

PART 1

Complete the following fill-in-the-blank exercises.

1. How well a family works together and meets any crisis depends on its

   _____ and _____.

2. A family of _____ is the family one is born into, and a family of

   _____ is one the person establishes.

State the terms that describe the types of families defined below. Indicate your answer in the space provided.

3. Parents may receive remuneration for their care; children in these families may

   feel very insecure: _____

4. Members related by social values, free choice-oriented, and/or may follow a charismatic leader: _____

5. Homosexual unions, and children may be added to the family by artificial insemination or adoption: _____

PART 2

List and describe the eight family tasks discussed in your text according to Duvall and Miller (1990).

1. _____

2. _____

3. _____

4. _____

5. _____

6. _____

7. _____

8. _____

■ Section Three: Critical Thinking for Application of Essential Concepts

PART 1

Circle the letter corresponding to the appropriate answer.

1. Which of the following would be representative of a National Health Goal related to achieving healthy family and community life?

   A. Maintain the baseline positive data for blood lead levels

   B. Work with families with financial management

   C. Lower the amount of physical abuse directed toward women

   D. Support gay rights activists

2. Which of the following describes family nursing?

   A. Concentrates on the family as the client

   B. Concentrates on the individual as the client

   C. Concentrates on the family point of view

   D. Concentrates on the individual's point of view

3. Which of the following is a characteristic of the single-parent family?

   A. Provision of support to family members as a common interest

   B. Involves reconstituted support and increased security

   C. Represents 50% to 60% of families with school-age children

   D. Temporary psychosocial comfort is provided by family resources

4. The nurse should identify the patterns of family life when selecting an intervention. Which of the following behaviors describes mobility patterns?

   A. Rapid perception of role change

   B. Less use of health care providers for health maintenance care

   C. Families who must choose between groceries and a child's immunization

   D. Sudden shifting of parental responsibility to one parent

PART 2: CASE STUDY

The nurse is counseling a family who is anticipating the adoption of a 6-year-old boy. The family is currently in the marriage stage of growth and development.

1. What rationale should the nurse use to formulate an approach when advising this family to visit a health care facility soon after the adopted child has arrived in the home?

2. How does the nurse explain why a larger percentage of adopted children may be put into a "high-risk" category for neurologic development?

3. What are some common factors that exist with parents who adopt children that may cause the parents to be less resilient when adjusting their lives to the presence of a new baby?

4. Why is it important for the adoptive parents to tell the child of his adoption as early as possible?

5. The adoption has been final for 6 months, and the family visits the community health center for a well-child preschool check-up. The parents state that the child exhibited defiant and hostile behaviors after being told of his adoption. How would the nurse analyze this behavior and give an explanation to the parents?

■ Section Four: Inquiry and Exploration

PART 1: CRITICAL INQUIRY EXERCISES

1. Identify a patient in your clinical setting and use the family assessment tool to identify the various systems in his or her community.

2. Use the results to create an ecomap (diagram depicting the relationship between the family and the community).

PART 2: CRITICAL EXPLORATION EXERCISES

Select a patient you are caring for in the clinical setting and create a nursing care plan for him or her, including an assessment of the family and community. State the nursing diagnosis found in making your assessment, and provide the appropriate nursing orders.

Sociocultural Aspects of Maternal and Child Health Nursing

CHAPTER OVERVIEW

Chapter 3 provides the student with a fundamental understanding of cultural differences and exercises to assist the student in identifying behaviors that are culture-specific while respecting the individuality of all persons. A case study is presented to assist the student in planning for nutritional support as it relates to culture. The critical thinking exercises include the formulation of a nursing care plan.

LEARNING OBJECTIVES

After mastering the contents of this chapter, you should be able to:

1. Describe ways that sociocultural influences affect maternal and child health nursing care.

2. Assess a family for sociocultural influences that might influence the way it responds to childbearing and childrearing.

3. Formulate nursing diagnoses related to culturally appropriate aspects of nursing care.

4. Develop outcomes to assist families who have specific cultural needs to thrive in their community.

5. Plan and implement nursing care that respects sociocultural needs and wishes of families.

6. Evaluate outcome criteria to be certain that goals of care related to sociocultural aspects have been achieved.

7. Identify National Health Goals related to sociocultural considerations that nurses could be instrumental in helping the nation achieve.

8. Identify areas of care related to sociocultural considerations that could benefit from additional nursing research or application of evidence-based practice.

9. Use critical thinking to analyze how the sociocultural aspects of care affect family functioning and develop ways to make nursing care more family-centered.

10. Integrate sociocultural aspects of care with nursing process to achieve quality maternal and child health nursing care.

KEY TERMS

acculturation	norms
assimilation	pain threshold
cultural values	pain tolerance
culture	stereotyping
ethnicity	taboos
ethnocentrism	threshold sensation
mores	transcultural nursing

■ Section One:
Identification of Key Terms and Concepts

Match the terms in Part a with the descriptions in Part B. Place the letter corresponding to the answer in the space provided.

PART A

1. _____ Culture

2. _____ Transcultural nursing

3. _____ Cultural competence

4. _____ Stereotyping

5. _____ Ethnocentrism

6. _____ Ethnicity

PART B

A. Individual perception that one's own culture is superior to all others

B. A view of the world and a set of traditions that a specific social group uses and transmits to the next generation

C. A cultural group into which one was born

D. Expecting a set of behavioral characteristics from a group of people without regard to their individual characteristics

E. The care of patients with cultural aspects as a guide to care

F. Integration of cultural elements to enhance communication

■ Section Two:
Short Answer and Completion Exercises

Complete the following fill-in-the-blank exercises.

1. The term _____ makes reference to people who speak Spanish as their

   primary language.

2. The _____ _____ looks upon making direct eye contact with

   another individual as a form of disrespect.

3. A physical examination that includes the assessment of the frontal and

temporal sinuses may be rejected by the _____ _____ because

they view the head as the seat of the body's _____ .

■ Section Three: Critical Thinking for Application of Essential Concepts

PART 1

Circle the letter corresponding to the appropriate answer.

1. Which of the following phrases best describes assimilation/acculturation as related to sociocultural differences?
   A. A demonstration of the most dominant family member's influences
   B. A loss of cultural expression as the customs of a dominant culture are taken on
   C. A family tradition practiced in future generations
   D. Placing "labels" on groups of people according to their ethnic backgrounds

2. Select the statement that best describes the nuclear family.
   A. A family consisting of the mother, father, and children
   B. A family consisting of the mother, father, children, and grandparents
   C. A family consisting of the mother, father, children, aunts, uncles, and cousins
   D. A family consisting of the mother or father and children

3. Identify the culture in which the oldest woman in the family is the dominant person in the family.
   A. Orthodox Jewish
   B. Chinese American
   C. Hispanic
   D. Native American

4. In the 1800s large numbers of immigrants came to the United States from many different countries and gave up their native country's traditions and values. Which of the following is the common explanation for the actions of these immigrants?
   A. Each culture found the American culture and beliefs to be equal or superior to their own.
   B. The immigrants feared the Americans and participated in the American culture to avoid cruelty and punishment.
   C. The immigrants joined the American "melting pot."
   D. Immigrants who did not take on the American culture were placed in lower socioeconomic groups.

PART 2: CASE STUDY

Tatiana Ochoa is a 30-year-old Mexican-American woman in her second trimester of pregnancy. She is visiting the clinic for a prenatal examination. The nurse finds that Mrs. Ochoa is anemic.

1. What approach will the nurse use to assess the source of Mrs. Ochoa's anemia?

2. What cultural practice related to nutrition may be responsible for the anemia?

3. What suggestions might the nurse offer to facilitate adequate nutritional intake to correct the anemia yet allow Mrs. Ochoa to assume the diet she prefers?

■ Section Four:
Inquiry and Exploration

PART 1: CRITICAL INQUIRY EXERCISES

1. As the head nurse of the ambulatory clinic, what principal understanding would the nurse need to have about the South Asian culture to give guidance to the staff members regarding how this population group responds to time-related events?

2. Collaborate with your classmates to create a mock nursing care plan for patients of this ethnic orientation who may be experiencing problems attending appointments or making the appointments on time.

PART 2: CRITICAL EXPLORATION EXERCISES

Some hospitals have taken an active role to include cultural sensitivity in the care of patients and their families. Research the hospitals in your area to identify those who have telephone service agreements to assist families with language interpretation.

UNIT II

The Nursing Role in Preparing Families for Childbearing and Childrearing

Reproductive and Sexual Health

CHAPTER OVERVIEW

Chapter 4 reviews the anatomy and physiology of the reproductive system. It addresses sexuality as it relates to each stage of growth and development in the lives of human beings. The nurse's role in providing sex education to children, adolescents, and adults is illustrated through teaching concepts in this chapter. A case study is included to provide research exposure on the current national health concerns and goals.

LEARNING OBJECTIVES

After mastering the contents of this chapter, you should be able to:

1. Describe anatomy and physiology necessary for reproductive and sexual health.

2. Assess a couple for anatomic and physiologic readiness for childbearing, biologic gender, gender role, and gender identity.

3. Formulate nursing diagnoses related to reproductive or sexual health.

4. Identify appropriate outcomes for reproductive and sexual health education.

5. Plan nursing care related to anatomic and physiologic readiness for childbearing or sexual health, such as helping adolescents discuss concerns in these areas.

6. Implement nursing care related to reproductive health, such as educating for menstruation.

7. Evaluate outcome criteria for achievement and effectiveness of care.

8. Identify National Health Goals related to reproductive health and sexuality and specific ways that nurses can help the nation achieve these goals.

9. Identify areas of care in relation to reproductive and sexual health that could benefit from additional nursing research or application of evidence-based practice.

10. Use critical thinking to analyze ways that clients' reproductive and sexual health can be improved for healthier childbearing and adult health.

11. Integrate knowledge of reproductive health and sexuality with nursing process to achieve quality maternal and child health nursing care.

KEY TERMS

adrenarche	gender identity	menopause
andrology	gender role	oocyte
anteflexion	gonad	perimetrium
anteversion	gynecology	premature ejaculation
aspermia	gynecomastia	rectocele
bicornuate uterus	heterosexual	retroflexion
biologic gender	homosexual	retroversion
culdoscopy	laparoscopy	thelarche
cystocele	lesbian	transsexual
dyspareunia	menarche	transvestite
endocervix	menorrhagia	vaginismus
endometrium	metrorrhagia	voyeurism
erectile dysfunction	myometrium	

■ Section One:
Identification of Key Terms and Concepts

PART 1

Match the terms in Part A with a definition or related statement from Part B. Place the letter corresponding to the answer in the space provided.

PART A

1. _____ Fallopian tubes

2. _____ Uterus

3. _____ Homosexual

4. _____ Mons veneris

5. _____ Clitoris

6. _____ Fourchette

7. _____ Biologic gender

8. _____ Pelvis

9. _____ Hymen

10. _____ Skene's glands

11. _____ Gender identity

PART B

A. Inner sense a person has of being male or female

B. Ridge of tissue formed by the posterior joining of the labia minora and the labia majora

C. Located bilateral to the urinary meatus; supplies lubrication to external genitalia during coitus

D. Finds sexual fulfillment with members of the same sex

E. Structure contains four parts: interstitium, isthmus, ampulla, and infundibula

F. A pad of adipose tissue located over the symphysis pubis

G. Term used to denote chromosomal sexual development

H. Serves to support and protect the reproductive and other pelvic organs

I. Accommodates the growing fetus during pregnancy

J. Elastic semicircle of tissue that covers the opening of the vagina

K. Small, rounded organ of erectile tissue at the forward function of the labia minora; sensitive to touch and temperature and is the center of sexual arousal

PART 2

Match the terms in Part A with a definition or related statement from Part B. Place the letter corresponding to the answer in the space provided.

PART A

1. _____ Semen

2. _____ Prostate gland

3. _____ Penis

4. _____ Vas deferens

5. _____ Spermatozoa

6. _____ Urethra

7. _____ Penile artery

8. _____ Epididymis

PART B

A. Primarily produced from the prostate gland

B. Conducts sperm from the testes to the vas deferens

C. Made of cylindrical masses, namely corpus cavernosa and corpus spongiosum

D. A branch of the pudendal artery that provides the blood supply for the penis

E. Carries sperm from the epididymis through the inguinal canal into the abdominal cavity

F. Produced in the testes

G. Anatomically located below the bladder; secretes alkaline fluids to protect sperm; accommodates the urethra as it passes through the center of the prostate gland

H. A hollow tube leading from the base of the bladder and passing through the shaft and glans of the penis

PART 3

Match the terms in Part A with a definition or related statement from Part B. Place the letter corresponding to the answer in the space provided.

PART A

1. _____ Masturbation

2. _____ Heterosexual

3. _____ Fetishism

4. _____ Celibacy

PART B

A. Finds sexual fulfillment with the opposite sex

B. Self-stimulation for erotic pleasure or sexual release

C. Abstinence from sexual activity

D. Sexual arousal by use of certain objects or situations

PART 4

Indicate if the following statements are true or false by placing a "T" or "F" in the space provided.

Mrs. Bell telephones the nurse in a well health care center because she would like information regarding ovulation. She states that she has a 28-day menstrual cycle and would like to know when she should expect ovulation to occur. In advising Mrs. Bell the nurse would know that:

1. _____ Ovulation occurs at the midpoint of the menstrual cycle.

2. _____ Basal body temperature is affected by the production of progesterone and is lowered just prior to ovulation.

■ Section Two:
Short Answer and Completion Exercises

State the terms for the following definitions. Indicate your answer in the space provided.

1. _____ Organ that produces sex cells

2. _____ Stage of life at which menstrual cycles cease

3. _____ Produced by adrenal cortex, testes, and ovaries

4. _____ Initiation of breast development influenced by estrogen

5. _____ Originating from the same embryonic organ

6. _____ The study of female reproductive organs

■ Section Three:
Critical Thinking for Application of Essential Concepts

PART 1

Circle the letter corresponding to the appropriate answer.

1. The nurse is counseling 11-year-old Mandy and her mother in an ambulatory health care setting. The mother is communicating concerns to the nurse with regard to anticipatory guidance about menstruation. Mandy has not reached menarche. The family appears receptive and interested about the importance of health care. The nurse would know that including menstruation as a part of health education on this visit would be important because

   A. menopausal changes that could be a threat to Mandy's health may be occurring.

   B. menarche should have occurred at age 9.

   C. Mandy is in jeopardy for experiencing regular cyclic hormonal changes.

   D. menstruation is considered to be an initiation to sexuality and womanhood.

2. Some couples experience sexual dysfunction during relations. When the female does not experience an orgasm because the male ejaculates before he desires, the dysfunction is referred to as

   A. dyspareunia.

   B. premature vaginismus.

   C. premature ejaculation.

   D. failure to achieve orgasm.

3. A condition that causes the female to experience pain during coitus, and is usually caused by endometriosis, vaginal infection, or hormonal changes, is called

   A. dyspareunia.

   B. premature vaginismus.

   C. sadomasochism.

   D. fetishism.

PART 2: CASE STUDY

As a summer student taking an independent study course, you are a mentor for a group of prospective college students. These students are matriculating in a post-high school program for persons pursuing health careers. To complete their curriculum, you must address the following principles of reproductive and sexual health.

1. State the primary role of the nurse in the promotion of reproductive health.

2. Describe four physiologic functions that explain how the activity of the hypothalamus influences the menstrual cycle.

3. Identify three environmental factors that may influence the preschooler's gender identity.

4. Summarize the physiological changes that occur in older adults that may alter the ability of both male and female to be sexually active.

5. Identify National Health Goals related to reproductive and sexual health and how the nurse may support the nation to achieve these goals.

■ Section Four: Inquiry and Exploration

PART 1: CRITICAL INQUIRY EXERCISES

Create a teaching plan to be used in a group setting for teenage girls. Describe how conception takes place using the sequel approach from the point of ovulation.

PART 2: CRITICAL EXPLORATION EXERCISES

Visit a public health department and assess the approach the nurse uses to teach about reproductive health care to patients who are requesting birth control measures for the first time.

Reproductive Life Planning

CHAPTER OVERVIEW

Chapter 5 discusses the methods available for reproductive life planning. These methods are presented with their physiologic actions and the impact on future pregnancies. The chapter examines the process of ovulation and potential side effects of an ovulation-suppressing agent. The principles of therapeutic communication when counseling the family who seeks health care on reproductive life planning are also discussed. Case studies are provided to assist the student in learning why specific methods of reproductive life planning are recommended over other available methods.

LEARNING OBJECTIVES

After mastering the contents of this chapter, you should be able to:

1. Describe common methods of reproductive life planning and the advantages, disadvantages, and risk factors associated with each.

2. Assess clients for reproductive life planning needs.

3. Formulate nursing diagnoses related to reproductive life planning concerns.

4. Identify expected outcomes for couples desiring reproductive life planning.

5. Plan nursing care related to reproductive life planning, such as helping a client select a suitable family planning measure.

6. Implement nursing care related to reproductive life planning, such as educating adolescents about the use of condoms as a safer sex practice as well as to prevent unwanted pregnancy.

7. Evaluate outcome criteria for achievement and effectiveness of care.

8. Identify National Health Goals related to reproductive life planning that nurses can be instrumental in helping the nation achieve.

9. Identify areas related to reproductive life planning that could benefit from additional nursing research or application of evidence-based practice.

10. Use critical thinking to analyze methods that could be used to promote reproductive health.

11. Integrate reproductive life planning with nursing process to achieve quality maternal and child health nursing care.

KEY TERMS

abstinence	fertility awareness
barrier method	intrauterine device
basal body temperature method	laparoscopy
calendar method	monophasic
cervical cap	natural family planning
coitus interruptus	reproductive life planning
condom	triphasic
contraceptive	tubal ligation
diaphragm	vasectomy
elective termination of pregnancy	

■ Section One: Identification of Key Terms and Concepts

Match the terms in Part A with a definition or related statement from Part B. Place the letter corresponding to the answer in the space provided. (Letters may be used only once; some letters will not be used.)

PART A

1. _____ Hypernatremia

2. _____ Menstrual extraction

3. _____ RU 486

4. _____ Isoimmunization

5. _____ Vasectomy

6. _____ Abstinence

PART B

A. Excision and blocking of the vas deferens to prevent passage of the spermato-zoa

B. Production of antibodies against Rh-positive blood

C. A result of an accidental injection of saline solution into a blood vessel

D. Blocks the effect of progesterone, usually administered with a prostaglandin

E. Removal of the uterine lining by suction or a syringe

F. Contraceptive method with a 0% failure rate

G. Suppresses ovulation and stimulates thick cervical mucus

■ Section Two:
Short Answer and Completion Exercises

PART 1

Complete the following short answer exercises.

1. List six side effects that may be experienced by the woman taking an oral contraceptive

   _____   _____

   _____   _____

   _____   _____

2. Describe three physiologic functions that suppress ovulation when "the pill" is used as a method of contraception.

   _____   _____

   _____

3. Describe how the "minipill" differs from the traditional oral contraceptive.

4. Discuss the use of IUDs, spermicides, and condoms by adolescents as methods of reproductive life planning.

PART 2

Complete the following table on methods of reproductive life planning.

Contraceptive	Description	Physiological Effect	Effect on Future Pregnancy
IUD			
Spermicides			
Diaphragms			
Condom			

■ Section Three:
Critical Thinking for Application of Essential Concepts

PART 1

Circle the letter corresponding to the appropriate answer.

1. A procedure using carbon dioxide and the coagulation and sealing of the fallopian tubes is called
   A. culdoscopy.
   B. laparoscopy.
   C. hysterectomy.
   D. minilaparotomy.

2. What day of the week after the start of menstrual flow should a woman begin taking an oral contraceptive?
   A. Sunday
   B. Monday
   C. Wednesday
   D. Saturday

3. When counseling an adolescent girl who expresses a desire to begin using the oral contraceptive method of reproductive life planning, it is highly recommended that the duration of her menstrual cycle be well established. How long should she have been experiencing menses before beginning to take the oral contraceptive?
   A. 1 year
   B. 2 years
   C. 3 years
   D. 4 years

4. Which of the following is thought to be a side effect of Depo-Provera?
   A. Thrombophlebitis
   B. Weight gain
   C. Excessive menstrual flow
   D. Osteoporosis

PART 2: CASE STUDIES

Friday, April 20, marks 1 week since Mrs. Nugent gave birth to a 6-pound, 7.5-ounce son. She has elected to use an oral contraceptive as her reproductive life planning method after his delivery. The physician prescribes an oral contraceptive to be taken for 21 days. Mrs. Nugent tells the nurse she is not clear about when to take her pills.

1. What instructions should the nurse give Mrs. Nugent on starting the use of this oral contraceptive?

2. How often should Mrs. Nugent take the pills, and when should she expect her menstrual flow to begin?

3. What are some suggestions that the nurse can offer Mrs. Nugent to help her remember to take her pill?

Ms. Jordan brings her 16-year-old daughter Tammy to the physician's office. Tammy experienced menarche 2 months ago and Ms. Jordan suspects she is sexually active. Ms. Jordan is requesting an oral contraceptive as a method for reproductive life planning for her daughter.

1. What permanent damage may occur if use of the oral contraceptive begins before the cycle is regulated?

2. Explain the relationship between oral contraception and the potential for alteration in skeletal growth with adolescent girls.

Mrs. Patterson, age 40, married and the mother of three children, is visiting the health care center to electively terminate her pregnancy at 8 weeks of gestation. She visits the community health care facility to be counseled on the procedure. As she is being examined, she asks the nurse if terminating her pregnancy would reflect negatively on her as a patient.

1. What are some very important guidelines that the nurse must remember when responding to Mrs. Patterson?

2. Mrs. Patterson is administered a laminaria for dilation of the cervix. Why would Mrs. Patterson be routinely placed on antibiotic therapy with this procedure?

■ Section Four: Inquiry and Exploration

PART 1: CRITICAL INQUIRY EXERCISES

1. Prepare a nursing care plan to provide health education and counseling for a patient who will be undergoing an elective tubal ligation. Focus on the future implications of the procedure.

2. Prepare a teaching plan for an adolescent who is pregnant and has expressed a desire to learn about contraceptives. The plan should address safer sex and a suitable method of reproductive life planning.

PART 2: CRITICAL EXPLORATION EXERCISES

1. Use the teaching plan that you constructed for the above exercise to teach a teen group in a community health care setting about safer sex and reproductive life planning.

2. Survey the retail market for condoms that are self-lubricated and treated with nonoxynol-9. Present your findings when counseling the adolescent in a clinical setting.

The Infertile Couple

CHAPTER OVERVIEW

Chapter 6 presents an overview of clients with fertility problems. The underlying physiologic and psychological bases for infertility problems are discussed. The use of the nursing process to address the needs of clients coping with infertility is explored.

LEARNING OBJECTIVES

After mastering the contents of this chapter, you should be able to:

1. Describe common causes of infertility in men and women.

2. Describe common assessments necessary to detect infertility.

3. Formulate nursing diagnoses related to infertility.

4. Identify appropriate outcomes for the infertile couple.

5. Plan interventions to meet the needs of the couple with a diagnosis of infertility.

6. Assist with interventions associated with the diagnosis of infertility or measures to promote fertility, such as health teaching.

7. Evaluate outcomes for achievement and effectiveness of care.

8. Identify National Health Goals related to infertility that nurses can participate in helping the nation achieve.

9. Identify areas of nursing care related to fertility that could benefit from additional nursing research.

10. Use critical thinking to analyze nursing strategies that can be used to support a couple through a fertility assessment.

11. Integrate knowledge about infertility with nursing process to achieve quality maternal and child health nursing care.

KEY TERMS

anovulation	primary infertility
cryptorchidism	secondary infertility
endometriosis	sperm count
erectile dysfunction	sperm motility
infertility	spermatogenesis
mumps orchitis	varicocele

■ Section One:
Identification of Key Terms and Concepts

Match the terms in Part A with a definition or related statement from Part B. Place the letter corresponding to the answer in the space provided.

PART A

1. _____ Anovulation

2. _____ Arborization

3. _____ Basal body temperature

4. _____ Endometriosis

5. _____ Infertility

6. _____ Laparotomy

7. _____ Secondary infertility

8. _____ Spinnbarkeit test

9. _____ Sterility

10. _____ Varicocele

PART B

A. The inability to conceive a child or sustain a pregnancy to childbirth

B. The stretching property of cervical mucus; indicates high estrogen levels

C. Introduction of a thin, hollow, lighted tube through the abdomen to examine the ovaries and uterus

D. A test for ovulation involving monitoring a monthly graph to determine when ovulation occurs

E. The inability to conceive because of a known condition

F. Enlargement of a testicular vein; may result in infertility due to venous congestion

G. Faulty or inadequate production of ova

H. Cervical mucus smear forms a fern pattern; occurs when high levels of estrogen are present in the body, as is noted during ovulation

I. The couple cannot conceive a child at present but has had a previous viable pregnancy

J. Implantation of uterine nodules to locations outside the uterus

■ Section Two:
Short Answer and Completion Exercises

PART 1

Complete the following fill-in-the-blank exercises.

1. A couple's reaction to receiving results confirming infertility may range from

_____ to _____ _____ to _____.

2. A _____ _____ is a woman who agrees to be impregnated by a man's sperm and carry the child for him and his partner.

3. _____ _____ would allow parents with X-linked diseases to limit passing the disease to male offspring.

4. _____ _____ is the instillation of sperm into the uterus to aid conception.

5. _____ _____ fertilization involves exposing an egg to sperm outside the woman's body and transferring the embryo to the woman's uterus.

PART 2

Complete the following short answer exercises.

1. Discuss measures a man can take to increase his sperm count.

2. Describe appropriate nursing diagnoses related to the impact fertility testing and news of infertility could have on the involved couple.

3. Discuss two benefits of childless living.

■ Section Three: Critical Thinking for Application of Essential Concepts

PART 1

Circle the letter corresponding to the appropriate answer.

1. Which of the following is true about fertility studies?
   A. Fertility studies should be undertaken more quickly with younger women.
   B. If a couple is very anxious about infertility, studies should not be delayed regardless of the couple's age.
   C. Initial testing involves only the partner suspected of infertility.
   D. Women under 30 years of age should be referred for evaluation after 6 months of infertility.

2. Diane has been told she has blocked fallopian tubes. Which of the following fertility options should the nurse help her to explore?

   A. Hormonal therapy

   B. Artificial insemination

   C. In vitro fertilization

   D. Gamete intrafallopian transfer

3. Practical suggestions to help achieve fertility would include which of the following?

   A. Having coitus every day will increase chances for fertility.

   B. Douching should be done before coitus to promote sperm mobility.

   C. The male-superior position for coitus is best to achieve conception by placing sperm near the cervix.

   D. The woman should ambulate immediately after coitus to mobilize the egg toward sperm.

PART 2

Determine if the nursing interventions described for each situation are appropriate or inappropriate. Indicate your answer by placing an "A" or an "I" on the space provided.

1. _____ Spend time alone with each client when helping a couple faced with infertility.

2. _____ Instruct a man to have intercourse 24 hours before the time the semen specimen is collected for analysis.

3. _____ Inform a woman that after a uterine endometrial biopsy, bleeding and clot passage are to be expected and will stop eventually.

4. _____ Assess a woman for allergy to iodine before she undergoes a hysterosalpingography.

5. _____ Counsel a man to wear warm, supportive underwear to heat the testes and increase sperm production.

PART 3: CASE STUDY

Marilyn and Palo Jaketes have been married for 3 years. For the past year they have had unprotected sex an average of three or four times per week in an effort to conceive. They have come to the clinic for assessment and counseling.

1. How might the ages of Mr. and Mrs. Jaketes affect their fertility evaluation and possible solutions for infertility?

2. What cultural beliefs might the Jaketes have that should be considered when discussing measures to facilitate fertility? How might cultural beliefs affect their choice of alternatives to childbirth?

3. What measures could you take to support the Jaketes through their emotional responses to news of infertility?

■ Section Four: Inquiry and Exploration

PART 1: CRITICAL INQUIRY EXERCISES

1. Prepare a teaching plan for an infertile couple that outlines various options.

2. When might adoption be an unacceptable option for a couple?

PART 2: CRITICAL EXPLORATION EXERCISES

Explore the facilities in your city to which you might refer clients with infertility problems (e.g., sperm or egg banks, infertility clinics, and adoption agencies).

UNIT III

The Nursing Role in Caring for the Pregnant Family

Genetic Assessment and Counseling

CHAPTER OVERVIEW

Chapter 7 presents an overview of basic principles and concepts related to genetic assessment and counseling. The inheritance of disease and types of genetic defects are discussed. The role of nurses in genetic counseling and the care of clients with genetic disorders are explored.

LEARNING OBJECTIVES

After mastering the contents of this chapter, you should be able to:

1. Describe the nature of inheritance and patterns of recessive and dominant mendelian inheritance and common chromosomal aberrations, such as nondisjunction syndromes.

2. Assess a family for the probability of inheriting a genetic disorder.

3. Formulate nursing diagnoses related to genetic disorders.

4. Establish outcomes that meet the needs of the pregnant family undergoing genetic assessment and counseling.

5. Plan nursing care related to an alteration in genetic health, such as assisting with an amniocentesis.

6. Implement nursing care related to identification of or counseling for a genetic disorder.

7. Evaluate outcomes for achievement and effectiveness of nursing care.

8. Identify National Health Goals and specific measures related to genetic disorders that nurses can take to help the nation achieve these goals.

9. Identify areas related to genetic assessment that could benefit from additional nursing research.

10. Use critical thinking to analyze ways that nurses can contribute to health education and counseling for genetic issues.

11. Integrate knowledge of genetic inheritance with nursing process to achieve quality maternal and child health nursing care.

KEY TERMS

alleles
chromosomes
dermatoglyphics
dominant gene
genes
genetics
genome
genotype

heterozygous trait
homozygous trait
imprinting
karyotype
meiosis
nondisjunction
phenotype
recessive gene

■ Section One:
Identification of Key Terms and Concepts

PART 1

Match the terms in Part A with a definition or related statement from Part B. Place the letter corresponding to the answer in the space provided.

PART A

1._____ Genetic disorder

2. _____ Chromosomes

3. _____ Phenotype

4. _____ Imprinting

5. _____ Homozygous

6. _____ Surrogate

7. _____ Dominant gene

8. _____ Polygenic inheritance

9. _____ Genetic marker

10. _____ Karyotyping

PART B

A. Identifies if chromosomal material has come from the male or female parent

B. Specific point on a chromosome marking the location of a missing or abnormal gene

C. A woman agreeing to undergo artificial insemination by the male partner's sperm and to bear a child for the couple

D. Material of heredity; strands of genes in the nucleus of body cells

E. When paired with other genes, these genes will always be expressed.

F. Can be passed from one generation to the next

G. Visual inspection of the chromosome pattern

H. Having two like genes for a trait

I. An outward appearance or expression of the genes

J. Diseases tend to have a higher than usual incidence in some families than in others

PART 2

Match each disease/condition listed in Part A with its usual pattern of inheritance or cause listed in Part B. Place the letter corresponding to the answer in the space provided. (Letters may be used more than once or not at all, and some answers may require two or more letters.)

PART A

1. _____ Diabetes

2. _____ Huntington's disease

3. _____ Hemophilia A

4. _____ Down syndrome

5. _____ Cystic fibrosis

6. _____ Turner's syndrome

7. _____ Duchenne muscular dystrophy

PART B

A. Dominant inheritance

B. Recessive inheritance

C. Multifactorial inheritance

D. X-linked inheritance

E. Division defect

F. Deletion abnormalities

G. Translocation abnormalities

H. Mosaicism

I. Isochromosomes

■ Section Two:
Short Answer and Completion Exercises

PART 1

Complete the following short answer exercises.

1. Discuss the merits of genetic testing for a couple at risk for having a child with an incurable genetic disease.

2. Differentiate between the chance of inheriting a disease if both parents are heterozygous for the trait and the disease is dominantly inherited, and the chance of inheritance if the disease is recessively inherited.

3. Discuss two of the four main purposes of genetic counseling.

4. Discuss why genetic counseling might be ineffective after the diagnosis of the pregnancy or immediately after the birth of a child with a defect.

PART 2

Complete the following fill-in-the-blank exercises.

1. Genetic counseling will _____ a couple about the genetic disorder and the chances that their child might _____ it.

2. Health professionals have a _____ and _____ obligation to share genetic information with the involved couple and no one else.

3. Couples who undergo genetic counseling and are informed they have a genetic abnormality in the family and might have a child with a genetic defect might experience a loss of _____ _____. The nurse must offer _____ to help them deal with the feelings they experience.

■ Section Three:
Critical Thinking for Application of Essential Concepts

PART 1

Circle the letter corresponding to the appropriate answer.

1. If "large feet" is a recessive trait and one parent is heterozygous for the trait and the other parent is homozygous for the trait, what are the chances that a child of this union will have large feet?
   A. 25% (1 in 4)
   B. 50% (2 in 4)
   C. 75% (3 in 4)
   D. 100% (4 in 4)

2. Which of the following individuals must be heterozygous for the recessive disease trait?
   A. Adam, who has no symptoms of the disease but has passed it on to his child
   B. Barbara, who displays no symptoms and has no children with the disease
   C. Peter, who has symptoms of the disease and has an affected child
   D. Wendy, who has symptoms of the disease but has no affected child

3. Which of the following couples would benefit most from referral for immediate genetic counseling?

    A. Tom, age 50, and Alice, age 42, who have just discovered they are going to have a baby

    B. Jim and Melissa, who have just had an infant with cystic fibrosis

    C. John and Jean, who want to have a baby but only want a male child

    D. Pete, who has hemophilia, and DeeDee, who have been married for a year and want to have a child

4. What role could the nurse play in genetic counseling?

    A. Assess the options available to a couple and select the best ones to present for the couple to choose from

    B. Inform the couple of the procedures they may undergo in genetic screening and in genetic counseling

    C. Instruct parents on the need for an immediate abortion if both persons have the trait for a dominant disease

    D. Limit the information provided to the couple about the genetic defect to avoid influencing their decision

5. To determine if a disorder occurred by chance or is carried by family members, a nurse should collect which of the following data?

    A. A history of the couple's sexual pattern during the time of conception

    B. As complete a family history of infant deaths or abnormalities as possible

    C. A prenatal history of nausea and reports of back pain in the last trimester

    D. Physical assessment of the infant's eye and hair color

6. The nurse should explain to the couple undergoing a genetic screening that Barr body determination is helpful to do which of the following?

    A. Allow visualization of an individual's chromosome pattern

    B. Detect chromosomal defects through chorionic villi sampling

    C. Determine the sex of an individual with ambiguous (unclear) genitalia

    D. Provide an analysis of the amniotic fluid and the fetal acid—base balance

7. Nursing measures that may be implemented when preparing a woman for amniocentesis should include which of the following?

    A. Determine that the woman is in her fifth to eighth week of pregnancy.

    B. Discuss the 10% risk of premature labor being stimulated.

    C. Support the woman who is beginning to accept the pregnancy and bond with the fetus.

    D. Explain that the procedure involves scanning with no invasive measures.

8. Which of the following would be a viable option for a couple found to be at high risk for producing a child with an inherited disease or defect?

    A. Delivery through cesarean section instead of vaginal delivery

    B. Implantation of a donor embryo if the female has the inherited trait

    C. Repair of fetal defects outside the uterus after fertilization

    D. Using the Lamaze method, which would reduce the risk of defects

PART 2: CASE STUDY

Bell and Bennie Johnson, both 32 years old, have been married for 1 year and want to have a baby. Bell has come for a complete physical and states she's concerned that she is too old for a healthy pregnancy. While doing the history, the nurse discovers Bell has a brother with Duchenne muscular dystrophy (DMD).

1. What is the significance of X-linked inheritance in determining the chances that Bell will have a baby with DMD if Bell is a carrier?

2. If Bell gives birth to a child with DMD, what nursing actions would be appropriate to help Bennie and Bell in planning for the future needs of their family and the child? Would it be appropriate for the nurse to approach family members, explain the genetic defect, and encourage them to support the couple? Why or why not?

■ Section Four:
Inquiry and Exploration

PART 1: CRITICAL INQUIRY EXERCISES

1. Write a brief statement on your opinion regarding the use of amniocentesis to determine if a fetus is without defects and if the couple should continue or terminate the pregnancy.

2. How might testing to determine the gender of an infant become an ethical dilemma? What are your thoughts regarding the use of modern technology to determine the gender of a child when a gender-specific genetic disorder is possible? When no disorder is likely?

PART 2: CRITICAL EXPLORATION EXERCISES

Attend a genetic counseling session and write a short report on the content discussed and reactions noted from the couple.

CHAPTER 8

The Growing Fetus

CHAPTER OVERVIEW

The development of the fetus is a complex phenomenon that originates from the union of an ovum and a sperm. When united, the ovum and the sperm form a single cell called the zygote. This chapter allows the student to explore all the stages of fetal development, enabling him or her to help the childbearing family understand the changes that take place during pregnancy. The student is also challenged to learn nursing principles necessary to conduct fetal monitoring and convey findings to the members of the childbearing family.

LEARNING OBJECTIVES

After mastering the contents of this chapter, you should be able to:

1. Describe the growth and development of the fetus by gestation week.

2. Assess fetal growth and development through maternal and pregnancy landmarks.

3. Formulate nursing diagnoses related to the needs of the pregnant woman and developing fetus.

4. Establish outcome criteria that meet the needs of the growing fetus.

5. Plan nursing care that promotes healthy fetal growth.

6. Implement nursing care to help ensure a safe pregnancy outcome and a safe fetal environment.

7. Evaluate expected outcomes for achievement and effectiveness of care.

8. Identify National Health Goals related to fetal growth that nurses can help the nation to achieve.

9. Identify areas of fetal health that could benefit from additional nursing research or application of evidence-based practice.

10. Use critical thinking to analyze ways to promote fetal growth and development.

11. Integrate knowledge of fetal growth and development with nursing process to achieve quality maternal and child health nursing care.

KEY TERMS

amniocentesis	ductus venosus	morula
amniotic cavity	ectoderm	neural plate
amniotic membrane	embryo	nonstress test
blastocyst	entoderm	oligohydramnios
cephalocaudal	expected date of birth	organogenesis
chorionic membrane	fertilization	quickening
chorionic villi	fetoscopy	surfactant
coelocentesis	fetus	trophoblast
corona radiata	foramen ovale	umbilical cord
cotyledons	hydramnios	Wharton's jelly
decidua basalis	implantation	yolk sac
decidua capsularis	lightening	zona pellucida
decidua vera	McDonald's rule	zygote
ductus arteriosus	mesoderm	

▪ Section One:
Identification of Key Terms and Concepts

Match the terms in Part A with a definition or related statement from Part B. Place the letter corresponding to the answer in the space provided.

PART A

✓ 1. __G__ Implantation

2. __D__ Amniocentesis – aspiration of amniotic fluid fr. preg. uterus for exam

3. __J__ Surfactant – a phospholipid substance that decreases alveolar surface tension on expiration

4. __A__ Decidua – 3 part organ (basalis, capsularis, vera) discarded following birth

5. __I__ Umbilical cord

6. __E__ McDonald's rule

7. __H__ Wharton's jelly

8. __B__ Human chorionic gonadotropin

9. __F__ Cephalocaudal

10. __C__ Coelocentesis – transvaginal aspiration of fluid that collects in the extraembry. cavity in early pregnancy

PART B

A. Three-part organ (basalis, capsularis, and vera) that is discarded following the birth of a child

B. Hormone found in the bloodstream shortly after conception and prior to first missed menstrual period

C. Transvaginal aspiration of fluid that collects in the extraembryonic cavity in early pregnancy

D. Aspiration of amniotic fluid from the pregnant uterus for examination

E. A method of determining that the fetus is growing in utero by measuring fundal (uterine) height

F. Developmental pattern (head-to-tail)

G. Contact between the blastocyst and the uterine endothelium occurring approximately 8 to 10 days after fertilization

H. A gelatinous mucopolysaccharide that gives the umbilical cord body and prevents pressure on the vein and arteries

I. Functions to transport oxygen and nutrients to the fetus from the placenta and to return waste products from the fetus to the placenta

J. A phospholipid substance that decreases alveolar surface tension on expiration

■ Section Two: Short Answer and Completion Exercises

PART 1

Using the weeks of gestational ages, identify the major milestones of fetal development.

Gestation Period	Fetal Development Milestones
End of 4 gestation weeks	Spinal cord has formed and fused at the midpoint; arms and legs are bud-like; weight is 400 mg
End of 8 gestation weeks	extremities have developed, heart beating rhythmic.
End of 12 gestation weeks	20g. Sex can be determined nail beds forming 45g
End of 16 gestation weeks	55-120g ∓HR is heard c̄ ord. stethoscope, Lanugo
End of 20 gestation weeks	- sleep pattern, 223g, fetal movements felt; meconium upper intst.
End of 24 gestation weeks	550g, eyebrows + lashes, eyelids open
End of 28 gestation weeks	1200g, lung aveoli mature, testes begin to descent
End of 32 gestation weeks	1660g - aware of sounds
End of 36 gestation weeks	1800g - turn to head down
End of 40 gestation weeks	3000g (7-7.5lb) kicks actively

PART 2

Complete the following short answer exercise.

1. Explain how nutrients are exchanged from the mother to the fetus during pregnancy.

   through the placenta

   selecta osmosis through chorionic villi.

■ Section Three:
Critical Thinking for Application of Essential Concepts

PART 1

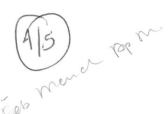

Circle the letter corresponding to the appropriate answer.

1. Beverly is being seen on her <u>first prenatal visit</u> at the health care clinic in her community. She reports that the first day of her last menstrual period was May 7, 2002. As calculated by Nagele's rule, Beverly's EDC will be

   A. New Year's Day 2003 (1-1-03).

   B. Valentine's Day 2003 (2-14-03).

   C. Veterans Day 2003 (11-12-03).

   D. April Fool's Day 2003 (4-1-03).

2. Mr. and Mrs. Mitchell are expecting their first child. On their visit to the physician's office for a scheduled appointment, they are jubilant over the pregnancy and curious about the health care procedures. As the nurse prepares Mrs. Mitchell for her assessment, she uses the Doppler to listen for the fetal heart tone. The nurse will expect the heart tone to be in a normal range of

   A. 110 to 120.

   B. 120 to 160.

   C. 170 to 180.

   D. 180 to 200.

3. The doctor has instructed the nurse to prepare Mrs. Mitchell for an ultrasound. Which of the following actions would be appropriate to prepare Mrs. Mitchell for this procedure?

   A. Instruct the patient to empty her bladder.

   B. Instruct the patient to drink an 8-ounce glass of water every 15 minutes for 90 minutes before the procedure.

   C. Shave the patient's abdomen.

   D. Place the patient in semi-Fowler's position with legs elevated.

4. Mr. Mitchell asks the nurse to explain why his wife needed an ultrasound. The nurse would respond appropriately by stating:

   A. "An ultrasound is a routine examination to monitor how the infant is growing and moving and to check for any complications."

   B. "The ultrasound test is used to measure the length and weight of your baby and to detect any chromosome abnormalities."

   C. "The ultrasound test is given to every pregnant woman. The explanation for why the test is given is complicated, but we will certainly let you know if the results are abnormal."

   D. "The doctor will explain the test to you, but I can tell you that we are checking to see if there are any problems with the pregnancy."

✓5. Mrs. Morrell complained of discomfort after having had an amniocentesis procedure. She is at 20 weeks' gestation and is 45 years old. Which of the following symptoms would prompt immediate action?

A. Lab results reveal abnormal chromosome cells.

B. Amniotic fluid contains fetal urine.

(C.) Mrs. Morrell describes symptoms of vaginal bleeding.

D. Mrs. Morrell describes symptoms of Braxton Hicks contractions.

PART 2: CASE STUDY

Mrs. Menendez is 44 years of age and at 28 weeks' gestation. She is admitted to the hospital after experiencing acute abdominal pain for several days. The physician orders a biophysical profile procedure to determine the well-being of the fetus.

1. How many parameters are to be considered in the biophysical profile?

✓ 6

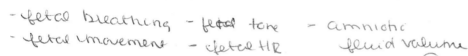
- fetal breathing - fetal tone - amniotic
- fetal movement - fetal HR   fluid volume

2. What is the highest potential score for each parameter? 8-10 (2)

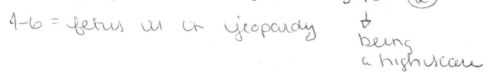
4-6 = fetus is in jeopardy   ↓
                                  being
                                  a high score!

3. Explain the reliability of the biophysical profile as an assessment tool.

4. How are the assessment findings used to determine the criteria score?

5. What major roles does the nurse play in obtaining the information for a biophysical profile?

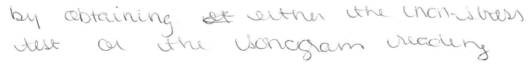
by obtaining either the non-stress test or the sonogram reading

■ Section Four: Inquiry and Exploration

PART 1: CRITICAL INQUIRY EXERCISES

1. Construct a diagram to illustrate how a couple may use the woman's body metabolic temperature as an indicator to predict ovulation. Demonstrate how coitus occurring 1 to 2 days before ovulation, as well as after ovulation, can result in fertilization.

2. Use colorful markers to draw a diagram of fetal circulation. Ask your instructor to allot you a portion of your laboratory class time to present your diagram. Name all anatomical structures of fetal circulation and discuss their functions.

PART 2: CRITICAL EXPLORATION EXERCISES

Formulate a nursing care plan expected outcome that addresses adequate fetal oxygenation throughout gestation. Then visit a health clinic on a day that several prenatal patients are scheduled to be seen. Note all of the implementations and procedures of the health care provider that can be viewed as actions to accomplish your goal.

Psychological and Physiologic Changes of Pregnancy

CHAPTER OVERVIEW

Chapter 9 addresses the psychological and physical changes a woman and her partner undergo during pregnancy. Though the physiologic changes of pregnancy are dynamic and extensive, they are considered an extension of normal physiology. The nurse uses this concept when preparing teaching plans and developing care plans. At the completion of this chapter the student will be knowledgeable about the interplay of these changes. This will enable the student to understand how to promote pregnancy as an extension of wellness in the family and throughout the pregnancy and early parenthood.

LEARNING OBJECTIVES

After mastering the contents of this chapter, you should be able to:

1. Describe common psychological and physiologic changes that occur with pregnancy, the underlying principles for these changes, and the relationship of the changes to pregnancy diagnosis.

2. Assess a woman for the psychological and physical changes that occur with pregnancy through health history and physical examination.

3. Formulate nursing diagnoses related to the psychological and physical changes of pregnancy.

4. Identify outcome criteria for the family's psychological and physical adaptation to pregnancy.

5. Plan nursing care related to the changes and diagnosis of pregnancy, such as helping women plan to get adequate rest.

6. Implement nursing care, such as health teaching related to the expected changes of pregnancy.

7. Evaluate outcome criteria for the achievement and effectiveness of care.

8. Identify National Health Goals that nurses could be instrumental in helping the nation achieve.

9. Identify areas of nursing care related to the psychological and physiologic changes of pregnancy that could benefit from additional nursing research.

10. Use critical thinking to analyze how the physical and psychological changes of pregnancy affect family functioning, and develop ways to make nursing care more family-centered.

11. Integrate knowledge of the psychological and physiologic changes in pregnancy with nursing process to achieve quality maternal and child health nursing care.

KEY TERMS

ballottement
Braxton Hicks contractions
Chadwick's sign
couvade syndrome
diastasis
Goodell's sign
Hegar's sign
hyperptyalism
lightening
melasma

Montgomery's tubercles
multipara
operculum
polyuria
positive signs of pregnancy
presumptive signs of pregnancy
primigravida
probable signs of pregnancy
pseudoanemia
striae gravidarum

■ Section One: Identification of Key Terms and Concepts

Match the signs and symptoms listed in Part A to the correct indication of pregnancy in Part B.

PART A

1. __B__ Positive test for hCG hormone in urine

2. __C__ Palpation of fetal movements

3. __C__ Quickening A

4. __B__ Chadwick's sign

5. __A__ Striae gravidarum

6. __P__ Auscultation of fetal heart sounds

7. __P__ Fetal outline felt by examiner B

8. __A__ Breast changes

9. __C__ Braxton Hicks contractions B

10. __C__ Sonographic fetal gestational sac B

11. __C__ Ballottement B

PART B

A. Presumptive
B. Probable
C. Positive

presum = maybe
prob = most likely
pos = ✓

■ Section Two:
Short Answer and Completion Exercises

PART 1

Complete the following short answer exercises.

1. What can the nurse do to help achieve the National Health Goals for women during pregnancy?

   by providing preconception counselling ....

2. You are caring for a pregnant client in the third trimester. What is one reason why you would advise her to lie in the lateral recumbent position while sleeping?

   so the fetus does not flatter the in vena cava causing a decrease in blood flow
   — also assists kidney to function @ best

3. What explanation would the nurse give to an expectant mother who has glucose in her urine but has tested negative for gestational diabetes?

4. Explain why it is important that pregnancy be diagnosed as early as possible and how this diagnosis may affect the woman's lifestyle and health status.

PART 2

State at least two physiologic changes in the following body systems that are sequelae to pregnancy.

1. Gastrointestinal system   *peristalsis - may set constipation*

2. Urinary system   *increas by 1500mL*   *frequent*

3. Skeletal system   *lordosis*

4. Endocrine system

5. Respiratory system   *diaphragm is flatten*
   making it hard to breath

■ Section Three:
Critical Thinking for Application of Essential Concepts

PART 1

Circle the letter corresponding to the appropriate answer.

1. Helga, age 14, is pregnant with her first child. She is in her second trimester and complains of problems with drooling. You would explain that

    A. she should be admitted to the hospital to assess the cause of this unusual symptom.

    B. this symptom shows a deficiency of sodium and indicates she should increase her salt intake.

    C. drooling is the body's way of eliminating excess fluid to prevent high blood pressure.

    D. the drooling is called "hyperptyalism" and is due to her increased hormone levels.

2. John, age 33, has just found out his girlfriend Ceilie is 4 months pregnant. Which of the following might indicate that a teaching plan is needed?

    A. John has not expressed pleasure or displeasure regarding the pregnancy.

    B. John refers to the fetus as "it" when talking to Ceilie about the pregnancy.

    C. John expresses great concern that if Ceilie should breastfeed she will ruin her figure.

    D. John says he hopes Ceilie will exercise more so she might have an easy vaginal delivery.

3. Which of the following is a correct example of the psychological tasks performed during the trimester discussed?

    A. During the first trimester women begin "nest-building" activities.

    B. In the second trimester women experience "quickening," which contributes to acceptance of the baby.

    C. During the third trimester the father-to-be usually begins the process of accepting the pregnancy.

    D. During the first trimester the father-to-be begins preparing for parenthood.

4. Which of the following is a positive example of reworking developmental tasks?

    A. The father-to-be begins to fantasize about being a carefree bachelor.

    B. An adolescent mother-to-be states she understands why her mother made her come home before dark.

    C. The father-to-be states his partner doesn't care for him since her pregnancy.

    D. A 42-year-old mother-to-be role-plays life before pregnancy.

✓5. Which of the following might indicate a problem in adjustment to pregnancy?

    (A.) A pregnant woman whose mother was abusive to her refuses to think about or discuss it.

    B. The pregnant woman reports an increase in sexual desire and greater enjoyment of sex.

    C. The father-to-be reports that his pregnant wife has frequent mood swings.

    D. The pregnant woman shows difficulty making decisions at work and at home.

PART 2: CASE STUDY

Dove Whitewater, age 44, has come to the clinic for a pregnancy test. She is alone, appears very anxious, and has an obvious swelling around her abdominal area. She states she has been nauseous for the past 5 months and usually eats only a light lunch since food makes her sick in the morning and at night.

1. What emotions might Dove reveal when her pregnancy is confirmed?

2. What are some taboos, or prescriptive and restrictive beliefs, held by some American Indians that would be physically harmless if followed by Dove during her pregnancy?

3. Dove states she might decide to terminate her pregnancy. What would your response be?

■ Section Four: Inquiry and Exploration

PART 1: CRITICAL INQUIRY EXERCISES

1. Develop a teaching plan that would give anticipatory guidance with reference to the acceptance of pregnancy. How might this plan be different for a single woman than for a married woman?

2. Explain how some psychological changes of pregnancy can be caused or aggravated by the physiologic changes of pregnancy.

PART 2: CRITICAL EXPLORATION EXERCISES

1. Perform assessments on three pregnant women in the first, second, and third trimesters. Record findings from your interviews that describe the psychological tasks of accepting the pregnancy, accepting the baby, and preparing for parenthood.

2. Assess a client in the second trimester of pregnancy who is experiencing Braxton Hicks contractions. Explain the differences between these and labor contractions.

CHAPTER 10

Assessing Fetal and Maternal Health: The First Prenatal Visit

CHAPTER OVERVIEW

When a woman visits a health care facility for the first prenatal visit, an assertive effort should be made by the health care providers to validate the pregnancy, determine the woman's health status and risk for complications, and initiate strategies that will encourage the woman and her family to establish positive behavior patterns of health promotion during the pregnancy and throughout their lives. This chapter allows the student to review the anatomic structures of the female body and demonstrate knowledge of how to appropriately intervene to provide nursing care, education, and guidance during the mother's pregnancy. A case study is included to help the student integrate therapeutic communication skills and nursing actions when assisting the patient with a pelvic examination.

LEARNING OBJECTIVES

After mastering the contents of this chapter, you should be able to:

1. Describe the areas of health assessment commonly included in a first prenatal visit.

2. Assess a pregnant woman's health status.

3. Formulate nursing diagnoses related to the health status of pregnancy.

4. Identify outcomes for achieving a healthy pregnancy.

5. Plan nursing care such as preparing a woman for a pelvic examination or fundal measurement.

6. Implement nursing care such as establishing a risk score for pregnancy.

7. Evaluate expected outcomes related to fetal or maternal health for achievement and effectiveness of care.

8. Identify National Health Goals that nurses can be instrumental in helping the nation to achieve.

9. Identify areas of prenatal care that could benefit from additional nursing research.

10. Use critical thinking to analyze ways to ensure family-centered prenatal care.

11. Integrate knowledge of pregnancy health assessment with the nursing process to achieve quality maternal and child health care.

KEY TERMS

abortion
age of viability
chloasma
conjugate vera
diagonal conjugate
erosion
gravida
ischial tuberosity
lithotomy position

multigravida
multipara
nulligravida
para
primigravida
primipara
speculum
true conjugate

■ Section One:
Identification of Key Terms and Concepts

PART 1

*Indicate if the following statements are true or false by placing a "T" or "F" in the
space provided.*

1. _____ The cervical os is found to be round and small in a nulligravida client.

2. _____ The petroleum lubricant should be used on the speculum when viewing the cervix.

3. _____ When a client is infected with a *Chlamydia* infection, the vaginal mucosa appears extremely
    inflamed with a greenish-yellow discharge.

4. _____ A platypelloid pelvis accommodates childbirth with fewer difficulties than the other three types of
    pelves.

5. _____ The purpose of a prenatal visit is to establish a baseline of present health and minimize the risk of
    possible complications.

■ Section Two:
Short Answer and Completion Exercises

PART 1

Complete the following short answer exercise.

Define and describe the four types of pelves.

1. _____

2. _____

3. _____

4. _____

PART 2

Using the chart below, describe how three separate specimens are obtained for a Pap smear.

Specimen Procedure to Obtain Specimen

1. _____

2. _____

3. _____

■ Section Three:
Critical Thinking for Application of Essential Concepts

PART 1

Circle the letter corresponding to the appropriate answer.

1. A pregnant client has delayed her first prenatal visit. She visits the prenatal clinic only after she starts to experience edema of the feet and hands. The nurse takes a history and physical to begin Mrs. Barton's care. The client's response to one of the nurse's questions is, "This is my third pregnancy. I miscarried twice, the first time I was 8 weeks pregnant and the last time I was 26 weeks." The nurse correctly records Mrs. Barton's pregnancy status as

    A. Gravida 2 P. O A.1

    B. Gravida 2 P. 1 A.1

    C. Gravida 3 P. O A.2

    D. Gravida 3 P. 1 A.1

2. During the examination of a pregnant client, while lying in the lithotomy position the client complains of dizziness and nausea. What would be an appropriate nursing action to relieve the client's discomfort?

    A. Administering an antiemetic ordered by the physician

    B. Offering small sips of ginger ale

    C. Assisting to a side-lying position temporarily

    D. Discontinuing the examination

3. Diplopia was noted during the assessment of a pregnant client. This condition is described as

    A. elevated pigmentation of the skin.

    B. double vision.

    C. facial edema.

    D. gingivitis.

4. Which of the following injectable vaccines would be safe to administer to a pregnant client?

   A. Varicella

   B. Measles

   C. Mumps

   D. Polio

5. A pregnant client has been previously prescribed the following medications. Which medication is considered to be detrimental during pregnancy?

   A. Acetaminophen

   B. Accutane

   C. Penicillin

   D. Folic acid

6. The physician asks the nurse to make sure his pregnant patient's next appointment is scheduled correctly. The patient is in her 33rd week. Her next appointment should be in

   A. 1 month.

   B. 3 weeks.

   C. 2 weeks.

   D. 1 week.

PART 2: CASE STUDY

Mrs. Goldstein is scheduled in the prenatal clinic for a pelvic examination. She will need to be prepared for the examination of several internal and external reproductive organs.

1. What position should Mrs. Goldstein assume once she is on the examination table?

2. Name the instruments that the nurse should have available for the examination.

3. How may a support person be of assistance to Mrs. Goldstein?

4. If she is found to be positive for the HIV virus, what decisions might she need to consider?

■ Section Four: Inquiry and Exploration

PART 1: CRITICAL INQUIRY EXERCISES

1. Diagram the four types of pelves on a poster. Illustrate to your class how the anatomy of the pelvis may accommodate or hamper the fetus as it progresses through the birthing process.

2. Determine four assessment criteria that would reveal findings that could help determine that a pregnant woman is at high risk for the HIV infection.

PART 2: CRITICAL EXPLORATION EXERCISES

Visit a prenatal health care setting and select a patient in the third trimester of her pregnancy who has been counseled and diagnosed as having a pelvis incompetent for delivery. Use your diagram as a tool to help the family understand the information discussed during counseling concerning the structure of the expectant mother's pelvis.

CHAPTER 11

Promoting Fetal and Maternal Health

CHAPTER OVERVIEW

Chapter 11 provides an overview of nursing care related to health promotion during pregnancy and the prevention of fetal exposure to teratogens. The general self-care needs of the pregnant woman, as well as common discomforts encountered during pregnancy, are reviewed. The use of the nursing process to plan and provide appropriate teaching for the woman throughout pregnancy is explored.

LEARNING OBJECTIVES

After mastering the contents of this chapter, you should be able to:

1. Describe health practices important for a positive pregnancy outcome.

2. Assess a woman's health practices and concerns during pregnancy.

3. Formulate nursing diagnoses to promote a healthy pregnancy.

4. Identify expected outcomes to promote a healthy pregnancy.

5. Plan health promotion strategies to limit exposure to teratogens or reduce the minor discomforts of pregnancy.

6. Implement care to promote positive health practices during pregnancy.

7. Evaluate expected outcomes for achievement and effectiveness of health promotion.

8. Identify National Health Goals related to pregnancy care that nurses can help the nation to achieve.

9. Identify areas of prenatal care that could benefit from additional nursing research and the application of evidence-based practice.

10. Use critical thinking to analyze ways to promote individualized and family-centered prenatal care.

11. Integrate knowledge of health promotion strategies with the nursing process to achieve quality maternal and child nursing care.

KEY TERMS

Braxton Hicks contractions
cytomegalovirus
fetal alcohol syndrome
leukorrhea
organogenesis period

Sims' position
teratogen
teratogenicity
toxoplasmosis

■ Section One:
Identification of Key Terms and Concepts

*Match the terms in Part A with a definition or related statement from Part B. Place
the letter corresponding to the answer in the space provided.*

PART A

1. _____ Braxton Hicks contractions

2. _____ Cytomegalovirus

3. _____ Fetal alcohol syndrome

4. _____ Leukorrhea

5. _____ Palmar erythema

6. _____ Headache

7. _____ Radiation

8. _____ Modified Sims' position

9. _____ Teratogen

10. _____ Toxoplasmosis

PART B

A. Whitish, viscous vaginal discharge

B. May be caused by expanding blood volume that puts pressure on cerebral arteries

C. Any factor, chemical or physical, that adversely affects the fertilized ovum, the embryo, or the fetus

D. A protozoan infection spread through contact with cat stool

E. Involves lying laterally with abdomen on the bed and with top leg forward

F. A member of the herpes family that can cause extensive fetal damage

G. Includes an infant being small for gestational age, with mental retardation and characteristic craniofacial deformity

H. Occurs in early pregnancy, probably caused by increased estrogen levels

I. Uterine cramps that may begin at the 8th to 12th week of pregnancy

J. Should be avoided by all women of child-bearing age except during the first 10 days of a menstrual cycle

■ Section Two:
Short Answer and Completion Exercises

PART 1

Complete the following fill-in-the-blank exercises.

1. Assessment of the pregnant woman concentrates on screening for the presence

   of _____ in the pregnant woman's environment and any _____

   that might be occurring with the pregnancy.

2. The major interventions associated with health promotion during pregnancy involve _____.

3. Five discomforts experienced during the first trimester of pregnancy are

_____, _____, _____, _____, and _____.

4. Three environmental teratogens are _____ and _____ hazards, _____, and _____ and _____.

PART 2

Complete the following short answer exercises.

1. For each of the following activities, discuss one concept that should be discussed with the pregnant woman: bathing, breast care, perineal hygiene, dressing, sexual activity, exercise, sleep, and travel.

2. Discuss four signs of beginning labor.

3. Describe the five categories of potential teratogenic drugs (A, B, C, D, X).

4. Discuss two instructions the nurse should provide to a pregnant woman who will be working related to all jobs, jobs requiring standing or walking, and jobs that require physical exertion.

5. Discuss how maternal stress may have a teratogenic effect.

■ Section Three:
Critical Thinking for Application of Essential Concepts

PART 1

Circle the letter corresponding to the appropriate answer.

1. Bobby has been experiencing severe constipation during her eighth month of pregnancy. An appropriate goal or outcome criterion for Bobby would be to
   A. become accustomed to the constipation and accept it as unavoidable.
   B. consume a diet containing high fiber, fruit, and extra amounts of fluid.
   C. have a bowel movement every other day to avoid daily straining activity.
   D. refrain from taking her iron supplement since it probably caused the problem.

2. When planning a teaching strategy for a pregnant woman, the nurse should do which of the following?
   A. Give information about how the woman can manage the specific problems she identifies as relevant in her life.
   B. Omit information related to minor pains of pregnancy to prevent the woman from developing hypochondria.
   C. Provide all information to the woman in a group session with other pregnant women so she can have someone to discuss it with.
   D. During the first prenatal visit, teach a woman the care measures necessary for health promotion throughout the pregnancy.

3. Bonnie, 6 months pregnant, is commuting 2 to 3 hours by car to school for a 6-week session. The nurse should discuss which of the following with Bonnie about travel?
   A. Dangers related to wearing lap seatbelts during the early months of pregnancy
   B. Methods of relieving stiffness and muscle aches and improving circulation during the drive
   C. The importance of taking motion sickness medications to lessen the nausea from driving
   D. The need to call her doctor and drive home immediately if she experiences premature labor or any danger signs of pregnancy

4. Sheila, 7 months pregnant, reports feeling her heart skipping a beat sometimes. The nurse recognizes these as heart palpitations and sets which of the following goal criteria? Sheila will
   A. demonstrate moving slowly from one position to another.
   B. lie supine when sleeping to keep pressure on her vena cava.
   C. plan a diet menu that includes high vitamin C content.
   D. verbalize intent to limit fluids to lower her heart's workload.

5. Dee is in her second month of pregnancy and complains of abdominal pain. The nurse should respond in which of the following ways to this information?

   A. Encourage Dee to put strong direct pressure on her fundus and hold it for 15 minutes whenever she feels this pain.

   B. Inform Dee that abdominal pain is expected at this stage of her pregnancy and she should learn to adjust to it.

   C. Inquire about the specific nature and location of the pain Dee reported, since it could indicate a complication.

   D. Tell Dee to lie on her side at night to relieve the pressure on her intestinal tract and stomach.

6. Which of the following symptoms is less commonly noted in early pregnancy?

   A. Braxton Hicks contractions

   B. Frequency of urination

   C. Ankle edema

   D. Varicosities

7. Tina is a heavy smoker (two packs per day) and is pregnant. Which of the following measures undertaken by Tina would indicate that a teaching plan for her had been most effective?

   A. She limited her cigarette smoking to one pack per day during her last months of pregnancy.

   B. She decreased her smoking by two cigarettes per day until she had stopped completely.

   C. She stated she will smoke only filtered cigarettes while she is pregnant.

   D. She voiced understanding that she will use nicotine gum and stop smoking immediately.

PART 2: CASE STUDY

Ginene Varez, 31 years of age, visits your clinic for her first prenatal check-up. She is in her first trimester of pregnancy. She complains of skipping heartbeats, headache, and nausea, and states she is worried that the "tension" of her job as an accountant in a perfume factory will have a negative effect on her baby. Her blood pressure and pulse are in the normal range.

1. What would you explain to Ginene about a common physical change of pregnancy that has likely resulted in both the headache and heart palpitations?

2. What measures would you suggest to help Ginene reduce anxiety from her job?

3. If you prepared a teaching plan to help Ginene avoid teratogens, what assessments would you need to make regarding her treatment of the nausea she experiences, and her job environment?

■ Section Four: Inquiry and Exploration

PART 1: CRITICAL INQUIRY EXERCISES

1. Prepare a teaching plan for a working woman that addresses methods for maintaining adequate nutrition and rest.

2. What are some realistic ways a pregnant woman can minimize exposure to common teratogens in the environment?

PART 2: CRITICAL EXPLORATION EXERCISES

Observe the initial prenatal visit for women in each of the following age groups: 12 to 17, 25 to 30, and 35 to 40. Note the differences and similarities in instructions given regarding activities and rest, and nutritional needs.

Promoting Nutritional Health During Pregnancy

CHAPTER OVERVIEW

Chapter 12 provides an overview of the nutritional needs of a woman throughout pregnancy. The nutritional guidelines for pregnancy are reviewed. The use of the nursing process to plan and provide appropriate teaching related to nutritional health during pregnancy is explored.

LEARNING OBJECTIVES

After mastering the contents of this chapter, you should be able to:

1. Describe the requirements for healthy nutrition during pregnancy.

2. Assess a woman's nutrition during pregnancy.

3. Formulate nursing diagnoses related to nutritional concerns during pregnancy.

4. Develop expected outcomes to assist the pregnant woman to achieve optimal nutrition during pregnancy.

5. Plan health teaching strategies such as ways to increase iron and calcium intake to promote optimal nutritional intake during pregnancy.

6. Implement nursing care that encourages healthy nutritional practices during pregnancy.

7. Evaluate expected outcomes for achievement and effectiveness of nutritional care.

8. Identify National Health Goals related to nutrition and pregnancy that nurses can be instrumental in helping the nation achieve.

9. Identify areas related to nutrition and pregnancy that could benefit from additional nursing research or application of evidence-based practice.

10. Use critical thinking to analyze the effects of different life situations on nutrition patterns and ways nutritional health can be improved.

11. Integrate nutrition knowledge with nursing process to achieve quality maternal and child health nursing care.

KEY TERMS

body mass index
complete protein
Hawthorne effect
hypercholesterolemia
hyperplasia
hypertrophy
incomplete protein

lactase
obese
overweight
pica
pyrosis
underweight

■ Section One:
Identification of Key Terms and Concepts

Match the terms in Part A with a definition or related statement from Part B. Place the letter corresponding to the answer in the space provided.

PART A

1. _____ Complete protein

2. _____ Hyperplasia

3. _____ Incomplete protein

4. _____ Lactase

5. _____ Linoleic acid

6. _____ Obese

7. _____ Phenylketonuria

8. _____ Pica

9. _____ Complementary proteins

10. _____ Pyrosis

PART B

A. A fatty oil that cannot be manufactured in the body from other sources

B. Foods containing fewer than eight of the essential amino acids

C. An abnormal craving for nonfood substances

D. A food containing all eight essential amino acids

E. Fetal growth occurring early in pregnancy; an increase in the number of cells formed

F. Foods that when cooked together provide all eight amino acids

G. A burning sensation along the esophagus caused by decreased gastric motility

H. For a woman, weighing over 200 pounds, having a body mass index over 29, or being 50% above ideal body weight

I. The enzyme needed to break down milk sugar into glucose and galactose

J. An inability to convert an essential amino acid into tyrosine

■ Section Two: Short Answer and Completion Exercises

PART 1

Complete the following fill-in-the-blank exercises.

1. A weight gain of _____ is currently recommended as an average weight gain in pregnancy.

2. The _____ of the food eaten is just as important as the quantity of food eaten.

3. A pregnancy diet should never contain less than _____ calories per day.

4. Pregnant women who are vegetarians may lack vitamin _____, vitamin _____, and _____ in their diet.

5. Underweight women may need to increase their caloric intake by _____ to _____ calories above the calories ordinarily specified during pregnancy.

PART 2

Complete the following short answer exercises.

1. Discuss the relationship between maternal dietary intake and fetal growth and development.

2. What factors may cause a woman to have decreased nutritional stores during pregnancy?

3. Discuss two types of food that should be avoided in pregnancy. Why should these foods be avoided?

4. Indicate the sources of the following substances and their significance for the pregnant woman: protein, calcium, fat, folic acid, iodine, iron.

■ Section Three:
Critical Thinking for Application of Essential Concepts

PART 1

Circle the letter corresponding to the appropriate answer.

1. Bonnie, 3 months pregnant, has reported for her first prenatal visit. The nurse should instruct her to do which of the following?

   A. Eat foods rich in protein, iron, and other nutrients to provide an additional 300 calories each day.

   B. Increase her intake of carbohydrates-breads and sweets-to prevent protein metabolism.

   C. Eat whenever she feels hungry because her body will let her know when she needs nutrients and extra calories.

   D. Limit intake of amino acids to prevent development of diabetic ketoacidosis.

2. Which of the following measures undertaken by Dee would indicate that a teaching plan on nutrition during pregnancy had been effective?

   A. Plans a diet limiting protein intake to minimize metabolic waste during her last months of pregnancy

   B. Remains slim during the first 5 months of her pregnancy and small during the final months of pregnancy

   C. States she understands that, although she is obese, she should not diet to lose weight but should avoid eating empty calories

   D. Voices understanding that she should take over-the-counter vitamin and mineral preparations twice daily to supplement her diet

3. Pam is a 23-year-old single mother who has a 15-month-old and a 3-month-old who was premature; she had a miscarriage before the birth of her 3-month-old. Her diet history revealed that she likes to eat fish and chicken. Pam should be considered at nutritional risk because of her

   A. prior pregnancies.

   B. risky age group.

   C. single marital status.

   D. unusual food preferences.

4. A woman with phenylketonuria should do which of the following?

   A. Avoid pregnancy, since it would aggravate her condition.

   B. Avoid food restrictions of any kind during her pregnancy.

   C. Return to a low-phenylalanine diet before becoming pregnant.

   D. Increase her intake of phenylalanine if she will breast-feed.

5. Which of the following would be an appropriate nursing intervention to help a woman with nausea and vomiting maintain adequate nutritional intake?

   A. Advise her to take daily laxatives to stimulate peristalsis and food digestion.

   B. Encourage her to eat meals before going to bed, when nausea is less severe.

   C. Suggest she eat foods that are high in fat to increase caloric intake.

   D. Teach her to refrain from eating for at least 6 hours prior to bedtime.

PART 2: CASE STUDY

Ellen, age 16, is in her second trimester of pregnancy. She is at the clinic for her initial prenatal visit.

1. What are the most important initial assessments you would make before discussing nutritional needs with Ellen?

2. What nutritional intake behaviors do most adolescents exhibit that might make it difficult to promote adequate nutrition for Ellen and her fetus?

3. Compare the dietary instructions you might provide for a pregnant adolescent like Ellen with those for a pregnant woman over age 35.

■ Section Four: Inquiry and Exploration

PART 1: CRITICAL INQUIRY EXERCISES

1. Prepare a 24-hour recall history using your own nutritional intake. Assess your dietary intake for adequacy. What changes would be necessary if you were pregnant?

2. What are five common foods served at fast-food restaurants that could be eaten to meet nutritional requirements? What are five foods that would be poor nutritional choices for the pregnant woman?

PART 2: CRITICAL EXPLORATION EXERCISES

Perform a diet history on a pregnant adolescent woman and develop a teaching plan that addresses the nutritional needs of pregnancy.

Preparation for Childbirth and Parenting

CHAPTER OVERVIEW

Chapter 13 addresses the woman who is preparing for the birth of a child. Physical and psychological readiness is addressed in terms of exercises and psychological techniques for pain control. The nursing interventions during the laboring process in the various types of birth settings are presented. The chapter presents a case study that describes principles pertinent to providing guidance to parents who may choose to participate in an alternative birth method.

LEARNING OBJECTIVES

After mastering the contents of this chapter, you should be able to:

1. Describe common alternative settings for birth and preparation necessary for childbirth and parenting.

2. Assess a couple for readiness for childbirth with regard to choice of birth attendant, preparation for labor, and setting.

3. Formulate nursing diagnoses related to preparation for childbirth and parenting.

4. Identify expected outcomes for the couple preparing for childbirth and parenting.

5. Plan nursing care such as teaching exercises that are effective for strengthening abdominal and perineal muscles for childbirth.

6. Implement nursing care such as supporting a woman during labor by the Lamaze method of prepared childbirth or helping a couple select and prepare for an alternative birth setting, such as the home.

7. Evaluate outcome criteria for achievement and effectiveness of care.

8. Identify National Health Goals related to preparation for parenthood that nurses could be instrumental in helping the nation to achieve.

9. Identify areas related to preparation for childbirth that could benefit from additional nursing research or application of evidence-based practice.

10. Use critical thinking to analyze ways that birth can be made more family-centered through the use of expectant parents' prepared childbirth classes and alternative birth settings.

11. Integrate the principles of prepared childbirth with nursing process to achieve quality maternal and child health nursing care.

KEY TERMS

alternative birthing center	cutaneous stimulation distraction
birthing bed	effleurage
birthing chair	gate control theory of pain perception
birthing room	labor-delivery-recovery-postpartum room
cleansing breath	labor-delivery-recovery room
conditioned reflexes	Leboyer method
consciously controlled breathing	psychoprophylaxis
conscious relaxation	vaginal birth after cesarean birth

■ Section One: Identification of Key Terms and Concepts

Match the terms in Part A with a definition or related statement from Part B. Place the letter corresponding to the answer in the space provided.

PART A

1. _____ Imaging

2. _____ Dick-Read method

3. _____ Conditioned reflex

4. _____ Tailor sitting

5. _____ Squatting

6. _____ Bradley method

PART B

A. Increases blood supply to the lower limbs and stretches the perineum

B. A physical response prompted by hearing a word or phrase

C. Method of childbirth based on the belief that birth is a natural process that should include the husband during the entire birthing process

D. Includes "sensate focus" inhibiting sensory input from reaching the cortex of the brain

E. Positioning the feet flat on the floor while stretching the perineal muscles

F. Method of childbirth based on the premise that fear leads to tension, which leads to pain

■ Section Two: Short Answer and Completion Exercises

PART 1

State the terms that are described by the following phrases. Indicate your answer in the space provided.

1. _____ Beginning of breathing exercises with deep inhalations and exhalations

2. _____ Impeding impulses at the level of the spinal cord to prohibit brain perception

3. _____ Encouraging progressive breathing, including conscious relaxation

4. _____ Light abdominal massage in conjunction with breathing exercises

5. _____ Used with repetition to strengthen the floor of the perineum

6. _____ Prevention of pain during birth by use of the mind

PART 2

Identify the advantages and disadvantages for the following birth settings.

Hospital

   a. Advantages_____

   b. Disadvantages _____

Alternative birth center

   a. Advantages_____

   b. Disadvantages _____

Home birth

   a. Advantages_____

   b. Disadvantages _____

PART 3

Describe the physiology of the following techniques of the gate control theory.

1. Cutaneous stimulation_____

2. Distraction_____

3. Reduction of anxiety _____

■ Section Three:
Critical Thinking for Application of Essential Concepts

PART 1

Circle the letter corresponding to the appropriate answer.

1. What is an appropriate adjustment to make in the birth environment in preparation for the Leboyer method?

   A. Spray the birthing room just before delivery with insecticides to reduce the microorganism counts.

   B. Raise the temperature of the room slightly just before the birth.

   C. Keep the birthing room as cool as the hospital delivery room to reduce the chance of bacteria growth.

   D. Darken the room completely after the birth to lessen the impact of the environmental change on the newborn.

2. Effleurage, a technique used to displace pain, is described as:

   A. light abdominal massage.

   B. focusing on an object to block sensory input.

   C. the prophylaxis method.

   D. the psychosexual method.

3. In consciously controlled breathing methods, level 5 behaviors are defined as:

   A. slow chest breathing at a rate of 6 to 12 breaths/minute.

   B. chest panting shallowly and continuously at a rate of 60 breaths/minute or more (during strong contractions).

   C. pant-blow rhythm intermittently with forceful exhalations.

   D. light breathing and expanding the rib cage, at a rate of up to 40 breaths per minute (during transition contractions).

4. Which of the following behaviors will assist the pregnant mother to avoid orthostatic hypertension?

   A. Holding her breath while exercising

   B. Hyperextending the lower back

   C. Quickly getting up from the floor after exercising

   D. Rolling from side to side during exercise

5. Flexing the lumbar spine can relieve backaches during pregnancy and early labor. This exercise is called:

   A. Kegel exercising.

   B. pelvic rocking.

   C. squatting.

   D. pelvic tailoring.

PART 2: CASE STUDY

Mrs. Virion, age 22, is interested in delivering her baby at home.

1. What factors would cause a woman to be considered a good candidate for a home birth?

2. What is considered to be the main advantage of a home birth?

3. State the expected outcomes when teaching Mrs. Virion how to perform the following exercises: abdominal contraction, pelvic floor contractions, and pelvic rocking.

■ Section Four: Inquiry and Exploration

PART 1: CRITICAL INQUIRY EXERCISES

1. Develop a teaching plan for the techniques of perineal exercises. Include a proposed time schedule for implementing the exercises for a woman who works from 8 AM to 5 PM.

2. Outline the main features of the popular Lamaze method of birthing. What behavioral characteristics would you look for in the family who would be most appropriate for this method?

PART 2: CRITICAL EXPLORATION EXERCISES

1. Attend a prenatal class at a well-baby health clinic. Present an overview of childbirth methods and education principles; discuss the ultimate goal of childbirth. Then provide the names of some referral sources to the mothers so they may obtain more information on childbirth and parenting education.

2. Interview a couple who has recently become aware of their pregnancy. Discuss several alternative settings for the birth and emphasize the advantages and disadvantages of each.

High-Risk Pregnancy: The Woman With a Preexisting or Newly Acquired Illness

CHAPTER OVERVIEW

Chapter 14 provides an overview of various systemic conditions that can result in a patient assuming a high-risk pregnancy status. The effects of various physical illnesses on the woman and her fetus during pregnancy stages are discussed. The use of the nursing process to plan and provide care for the patient, the fetus, and the family involved in a high-risk pregnancy is explored.

LEARNING OBJECTIVES

After mastering the contents of this chapter, you should be able to:

1. Define high-risk pregnancy including factors that contribute to its development.

2. Describe common illnesses such as cardiovascular disease, diabetes mellitus, or renal and blood disorders that can result in complications when they exist with pregnancy.

3. Assess the woman with an illness during pregnancy for changes occurring because of the pregnancy.

4. List nursing diagnoses related to the effect of a preexisting or newly acquired illness on pregnancy.

5. Identify appropriate outcomes that will contribute to a safe pregnancy outcome when illness occurs with pregnancy (e.g., planning ways a woman can secure more rest).

6. Plan nursing care for the woman with an illness during pregnancy (e.g., teaching insulin administration to a woman newly diagnosed with gestational diabetes).

7. Implement nursing care for the woman when illness complicates pregnancy.

8. Evaluate expected outcomes to determine achievement and effectiveness of care.

9. Identify National Health Goals related to complications of pregnancy that nurses can be instrumental in helping the nation achieve.

10. Identify areas related to illness and pregnancy that could benefit from additional nursing research or application of evidence-based practice.

11. Use critical thinking to analyze ways that nursing care can remain family-centered when a preexisting or newly acquired illness develops.

12. Integrate knowledge of high-risk pregnancy and nursing process to achieve quality maternal and child health nursing care.

KEY TERMS

deep vein thrombosis	insulin pump
glucose tolerance test	megaloblastic anemia
glycosuria	orthopnea
glycosylated hemoglobin	paroxysmal nocturnal dyspnea
high-risk pregnancy	peripartal cardiomyopathy
hyperglycemia	proteinuria
hypoglycemia	sexually transmitted disease

■ Section One: Identification of Key Terms and Concepts

PART 1

Match the terms in Part A with a definition or related statement from Part B. Place the letter corresponding to the answer in the space provided. (Letters may be used only once; some letters may not be used.)

PART A

1. __E__ Functional heart murmur   C

2. __J__ Paroxysmal nocturnal dyspnea

3. __F__ Megaloblastic anemia

4. __A__ Left heart failure

5. __G__ Pyelonephritis   K

6. __H__ Hiatal hernia

7. __I__ Scoliosis

8. __K__ Systemic lupus erythematosus   G

9. __D__ Pseudoanemia   B

10. __L__ *Chlamydia trachomatis*

PART B

A. Occurs when mitral valve stenosis or insufficiency or aortic coarctation causes a decrease in cardiac output and back pressure to the lungs

B. A normal decrease in the red blood cell count due to the expanded blood volume of pregnancy

C. An innocent, transient escape of fluid through heart valves due to increased blood flow past valves that can occur during pregnancy

D. Hemoglobin levels below 11 mg/dL due to low iron intake

E. Occurs when pulmonary stenosis causes a backup of fluid into the vena cava and subsequent engorgement of the venous circulation

F. Low blood levels with enlarged red blood cells related to folic acid deficiency

G. A multisystem connective tissue disease that may result in acute nephritis

H. A portion of the stomach extended through the diaphragm that can result in inability to eat due to heartburn

I. Lateral curvature of the spine that may cause pelvic distortion that can interfere with childbirth

J. Sudden waking during the night with severe shortness of breath

K. Kidney infection that can result in premature labor or rupture of membranes

L. The most common vaginal infection seen during pregnancy

PART 2

*Match the terms in Part A with a definition or related statement in Part B. Place the
letter corresponding to the answer in the space provided.*

PART A

1. ___C___ Viral hepatitis

2. ___D___ Human immunodeficiency virus

3. ___E___ Schizophrenia

4. ___F___ Tonic-clonic seizures

5. ___B___ Burns

6. ___A___ Celiotomy

PART B

A. Exploratory abdominal surgery performed to detect bleeding due to traumatic
injury

B. Dangerous to mother and fetus due to carbon monoxide and fluid/electrolyte
losses

C. Antigens can be spread to the infant from breast milk

D. Maternal infection with this virus requires active interactions to reduce fetal
exposure to maternal blood

E. May need to be treated with teratogenic medication

F. Could result in anoxia from spasm of chest muscles

■ Section Two: Short Answer and Completion Exercises

PART 1

Complete the following short answer exercises.

1. List one example each of psychological, social, and physical factors that can
   cause a pregnancy to be categorized as high risk during the pre-pregnancy,
   pregnancy, and labor and delivery periods.

2. Describe how pregnancy can cause a woman to develop a urinary tract
   infection.

3. Discuss the key issues that should be included in a teaching plan for a pregnant woman who is a diabetic or who develops diabetes during pregnancy. Address diet, exercise, insulin, and glucose monitoring.

4. Discuss four common sexually transmitted diseases and name one effect each could have on a newborn.

5. Describe one safety precaution in each of three areas-home, work, and automobile safety-that may be taken by a pregnant woman to prevent accidental injury.

6. Describe the procedure for airway clearance on a pregnant choking victim.

PART 2

Complete the following fill-in-the-blank statements and chart.

1. ___poor___ ___placental___ ___perfusion___ could cause cardiac failure, anemia, and hypertensive vascular disease to result in fetal distress or low birthweight.

2. Three factors in pregnancy that can result in venous thromboembolic disease are _____ _____ _____ , _____, and _____ _____ _____ .

3. Indicate the effects the following respiratory conditions may have on the mother or the fetus, and note the appropriate treatment: nasopharyngitis, asthma, pneumonia, tuberculosis.

Condition	Fetal Effect/Treatment	Maternal Effect/Treatment
Nasopharyngitis		
Asthma		
Pneumonia		
Tuberculosis		

■ Section Three:
Critical Thinking for Application of Essential Concepts

PART 1

Circle the letter corresponding to the appropriate answer.

1. Melle, 12 years old, is 2 months pregnant and has a history of heart disease. Which of the following is true about her risk factors for high-risk pregnancy?

   A. Good nutrition and exercise will eliminate any added risk factors Melle may have for complications.

   B. Melle's heart condition will not affect her pregnancy, since she has not reached adolescence.

   C. Melle's youth will protect her from many problems experienced by older women with heart disease.

   D. Both Melle's age and heart condition will place her at risk for complications during pregnancy.

2. Which of the following could be included in the outcome criteria for a patient with the nursing diagnosis, "Knowledge deficit related to potential for altered tissue perfusion in fetus or mother related to maternal cardiovascular disease"?

   A. Bed rest is maintained at home after the 36th week of gestation.

   B. Fetal heart rate will remain between 120 and 160 beats a minute.

   C. Jugular vein distention is evident when lying at 45 degrees.

   D. Maternal blood pressure is maintained above 150 systolic.

3. When planning care for a pregnant woman with heart disease, the nurse should do which of the following?

   A. Assess all complaints of fatigue and note any accompanying dyspnea or pulmonary congestion.

   B. Discourage the mother from taking any medications during pregnancy, since they will affect the baby.

   C. Instruct the patient to eat as much food as desired to promote maximum fetal and maternal nutrition.

   D. Plan an exercise schedule to prevent thrombus formation during labor.

4. Which of the following interventions should be implemented with caution when caring for a postpartal woman who has heart disease or hypertensive vascular disease?

   A. Administration of prenatal vitamins

   B. Early ambulation with antiembolism stockings

   C. Encouraging bulk and high fiber in the diet

   D. Suggesting oral contraceptives as a birth control method

5. Pregnant women with venous thromboembolic disease

   A. are at risk for death from a pulmonary embolism.

   B. must have oral fluids restricted throughout the pregnancy.

   C. receive heparin as soon as their labor begins.

   D. should be taught to keep their legs crossed at the knee when sitting.

6. Patients with megaloblastic anemia should be encouraged to do which of the following?

   A. Avoid pregnancy, since they cannot carry the baby to term.

   B. Avoid excessive fluid intake, which has caused this hemodilution.

   C. Take over-the-counter multivitamins.

   D. Take the prescribed folic acid supplements.

7. When planning care for a pregnant patient with sickle-cell anemia, the nurse might establish which of the following outcome criteria? The patient

   A. lies on her back in a semi-Fowler's position when sleeping.

   B. rests with her legs elevated when sitting in a chair.

   C. reports intent to get a sickle-cell antigen shot after delivery.

   D. states understanding of need to limit fluid intake to 16 ounces/day.

8. Patients with chronic renal disease or who have had kidney transplants may have difficulty in pregnancy for which of the following reasons?

   A. Fetal waste products must be excreted in addition to maternal.

   B. Hormones released in pregnancy can cause rejection of transplant.

   C. Increased glomerular filtration rate causes decreased serum creatinine level.

   D. Steroids may cause excessive fetal growth stimulation.

9. Measures the nurse should implement for the pregnant patient with rheumatoid arthritis include which of the following?

   A. Discuss the woman's intent to breast-feed so that medications can be changed if necessary.

   B. Instruct the woman to increase her intake of aspirin 2 weeks prior to term to offset the decrease in corticosteroids.

   C. Encourage the woman to contact her physician for a higher dosage, if methotrexate is prescribed.

   D. Assess the patient each week to monitor for blood clots due to salicylate ingestion.

10. Teresa, who is at 20 weeks' gestation, has been diagnosed with acute appendicitis. She expresses concern that the doctor is going to perform surgery. The nurse could explain which of the following?

    A. Delivery of the baby during cesarean birth at this point would be safer than trying to complete the pregnancy.

    B. Since the appendix cannot be removed at this stage of the pregnancy without disruption of the pregnancy, an abortion is necessary.

    C. If she prefers, the doctor can delay removal of the appendix until later in the pregnancy.

    D. Peritonitis could result from rupture of the appendix and would be dangerous for both mother and child.

11. Which of the following evaluation data would indicate that the nurse's teaching plan for the pregnant patient with cholecystitis had been effective?

    A. Aching occurs only in the right epigastrium after eating.

    B. Jaundice and pain remain absent throughout the pregnancy.

    C. The patient prepares a menu that is fat-free.

    D. The patient reports ingestion of high-cholesterol foods.

12. Which of the following is an appropriate outcome criterion for the pregnant patient who has seizures as a result of childhood meningitis? The client:

   A. demonstrates ability to recognize the Moro reflex as an early indication of fetal seizures.

   B. requires no supplemental oxygen administration during convulsions.

   C. states understanding that her child is not certain to have seizures just because she developed the condition.

   D. refrains from taking anticonvulsant medications during the first trimester to prevent congenital defects.

13. A pregnant woman diagnosed with diabetes should be instructed to do which of the following to control her glucose level?

   A. Discontinue insulin injections until pregnancy is completed, since hormones will regulate glucose levels.

   B. Ingest a smaller amount of food prior to sleep to prevent nocturnal hyperglycemia.

   C. Notify the physician if unable to eat due to nausea and vomiting.

   D. Prepare foods with increased fat content to provide needed calories.

14. After delivery, a diabetic woman might need to do which of the following?

   A. Change to oral hypoglycemia agents, which will control glucose levels more effectively than insulin.

   B. Bottle-feed her infant, since insulin received through breast-feeding may cause hypoglycemia in the child.

   C. Refrain from taking insulin during the immediate postpartal period, since insulin resistance is gone.

   D. Take medications to decrease uterine hypertonicity if hydramnios was present during pregnancy.

15. Which of the following data would support a diagnosis of "Ineffective family coping, compromised, related to poor communication between partners or potentially abusive father"?

   A. The woman and her husband always report together for prenatal visits.

   B. The woman states concern that her baby may not have a good heartbeat because she "fell down recently."

   C. You notice that the woman wears a low-cut dress or blouse at each prenatal visit.

   D. Examination reveals that fetal heart tones and fundal height indicate the baby might weigh over 8 pounds.

16. When preparing for a postmortem delivery, the nurse should do which of the following?

   A. Begin the oxytocin drip and regulate slowly to aid vaginal delivery.

   B. Determine if the pregnancy is earlier than 24 weeks' gestation, since a young fetus will be more likely to survive.

   C. Obtain equipment necessary for immediate resuscitation of the newborn.

   D. Prepare a consent form, since the surgery cannot be performed without a consent.

17. Which of the following nursing interventions would be appropriate when caring for a pregnant patient who has the nursing diagnosis "Altered tissue perfusion related to blood loss through gunshot or stab wound"?

    A. Encourage a sitting position that will maintain pressure to abdominal organs and control bleeding.

    B. Prepare to administer antihypotension drugs, which will cause peripheral vasoconstriction and maintain blood pressure.

    C. Recognize that since pregnant women have higher than normal fluid volume, small losses of blood will have severe vascular effects.

    D. Position the patient in a side-lying position to decrease vena caval pressure.

18. Nursing measures implemented with a pregnant patient who has experienced trauma would include which of the following?

    A. Concentrating on controlling the patient's anxiety first and foremost.

    B. Monitoring for other signs of shock, since the patient's skin might not be cold and clammy.

    C. Positioning the patient on her back in reverse Trendelenburg's.

    D. Recognizing that a heart rate increase of 15 to 20 beats above the nonpregnant rate indicates hypovolemia.

19. Pregnant women should be taught to be careful to avoid accidental injury. They are prone to falls for which of the following reasons?

    A. Additional weight from pregnancy may disturb balance when walking.

    B. Fetal activity stimulates the nerves of the legs and causes weakness.

    C. High levels of hormones often impair judgment, resulting in reckless behavior.

    D. Increased adrenalin released during pregnancy causes women to move faster than usual.

PART 2: CASE STUDY

Melinda Jaffe is a 28-year-old mother of two, ages 5 and 3. Melinda is in for her second prenatal visit. She is 5 months pregnant and has a history of congestive heart failure secondary to valve disease from childhood rheumatic fever.

1. What is the most dangerous time in the pregnancy for a woman with heart disease? Why?

2. How might the fact that Melinda has two young children affect her risk for complications from her heart disease? What nursing interventions would you plan?

3. How might Melinda's risk of complications be different if she had had valve replacement surgery years prior to the pregnancy?

■ Section Four:
Inquiry and Exploration

PART 1: CRITICAL INQUIRY EXERCISES

1. What would be the major points you would include in a teaching plan for adolescents that addresses the effects of sexually transmitted diseases on a fetus or on an infant after childbirth?

2. In what way, if any, would your teaching plan differ for an insulin-dependent diabetic who became pregnant, and for a pregnant woman who developed gestational diabetes?

PART 2: CRITICAL EXPLORATION EXERCISES

While on a postpartal clinical unit, review the chart of a patient with diabetes. Note the prenatal history, course of the pregnancy for glucose regulation, any complications experienced, postpartal glucose control, and status of the newborn.

CHAPTER 15

High-Risk Pregnancy: The Woman Who Develops a Complication of Pregnancy

CHAPTER OVERVIEW

Chapter 15 discusses the complications that can occur during pregnancy and the effects these complications have on the woman and her family. The use of the nursing process to plan and provide care for the client and family under these circumstances is explored.

LEARNING OBJECTIVES

After mastering the contents of this chapter, you should be able to:

1. Describe complications of pregnancy that place the pregnant woman and her fetus at high risk.

2. Assess the woman who is experiencing a complication of pregnancy.

3. Formulate nursing diagnoses that address the needs of the woman and her family experiencing a complication of pregnancy.

4. Identify outcomes to minimize the risks to the pregnant woman and her fetus.

5. Plan nursing interventions to meet the needs and promote optimal outcome for the woman and her family.

6. Implement nursing actions specific to the woman who has developed a complication of pregnancy.

7. Evaluate outcomes for effectiveness and achievement.

8. Identify National Health Goals related to complications of pregnancy and specific measures nurses can take to help the nation achieve these goals.

9. Identify areas of nursing care related to high-risk pregnancy that could benefit from additional nursing research or the application of evidence-based practice.

10. Use critical thinking to analyze ways that nurses can help prevent complications of pregnancy.

11. Integrate knowledge of complications of pregnancy with nursing process to achieve quality maternal and child health nursing care.

KEY TERMS

abortion	HELLP syndrome	premature cervical dilatation
ankle clonus	hemolytic disease of the newborn	premature separation of the placenta
cervical cerclage	hydramnios	preterm labor
cervical ripening	imminent miscarriage	preterm rupture of membranes
chorioamnionitis	incompetent cervix	pseudocyesis
complete miscarriage	incomplete miscarriage	recurrent pregnancy loss
couvelaire uterus	isoimmunization	Rh incompatibility
eclampsia	missed miscarriage	spontaneous miscarriage
ectopic pregnancy	placenta previa	threatened miscarriage
erythroblastosis fetalis	post-term pregnancy	tocolytic agent
gestational trophoblastic disease	preeclampsia	

■ Section One:
Identification of Key Terms and Concepts

PART 1

Match the terms in Part A with a definition or related statement from Part B. (Letters may be used only once; some letters may not be used.)

PART A

1. _____ Placenta previa

2. _____ Isoimmunization

3. _____ Cervical cerclage

4. _____ Imminent miscarriage

5. _____ Erythroblastosis

6. _____ Abruptio placentae

7. _____ Pseudocyesis

8. _____ Late spontaneous miscarriage

9. _____ Eclampsia

10. _____ Gestational trophoblastic disease (hydatidiform mole)

PART B

A. An interruption of pregnancy (natural causes) occurring between the 16th and 24th week

B. A rare implantation of the fetus in the cul-de-sac of Douglas

C. Proliferation and degeneration of the trophoblast villi

D. Low implantation of the placenta

E. Pregnancy-induced hypertension, proteinuria, and cerebral edema with seizure

F. Purse-string sutures applied to prevent recurrence of premature dilation and fetal expulsion (loss)

G. Occurs when Rh-negative women are exposed to Rh-positive fetal blood

H. Premature separation of the placenta

I. Uterine contractions and cervical dilation prior to fetal viability

J. Manifested by vaginal bleeding without associated symptoms

K. Produces progesterone needed to maintain the decidua basalis

L. Hemolytic disease of the newborn

M. Amenorrhea, nausea, and enlargement of the abdomen occurring in a non-pregnant woman

PART 2

For each of the pregnancy complications listed below, indicate when it usually occurs with the letter "A" for first trimester, "B" for second trimester, and "C" for the third trimester.

1. _____ Placenta previa

2. _____ Spontaneous miscarriage

3. _____ Hydatidiform mole

4. _____ Abruptio placentae

5. _____ Incompetent cervix

6. _____ Ectopic pregnancy

■ Section Two:
Short Answer and Completion Exercises

PART 1

Identify the conditions described below.

1. _____ An unplanned interruption of pregnancy before the fetus is viable

2. _____ Pregnancy in which implantation occurs outside the uterine cavity

3. _____ Hypertension of pregnancy that involves hemolysis, high liver enzymes, and low platelet levels

4. _____ Hypertension of pregnancy with BP elevated 30 mm Hg systolic or 15 mm Hg diastolic above prepregnancy values

5. _____ Excessive amniotic fluid formation

PART 2

Complete the following short answer exercises.

1. Briefly explain why it is important to determine the week of pregnancy at which bleeding began to occur.

2. Contrast the symptoms noted by a woman with a normal pregnancy with those that may be noted by a woman with an ectopic pregnancy.

3. Explain the difference between placenta previa and abruptio placentae.

4. Discuss the use of heparin to treat disseminated intravascular coagulation.

5. Explain how a teaching plan for a patient with multiple gestation would differ from a plan for a patient with single gestation in the following areas: activity, nutrition, complications, and role changes.

■ Section Three: Critical Thinking for Application of Essential Concepts

PART 1

Circle the letter corresponding to the appropriate answer.

1. Mrs. Dean is 2 months pregnant and has a history of two spontaneous miscarriages. Which of the following assessments indicates a potential for a third miscarriage?
   A. Lab results revealing an elevation in protein-bound iodine
   B. Dietary intake indicating 300 more calories than eaten by the nonpregnant female
   C. Reports of exposure to a child with rubella over a period of time
   D. Nervous, anxious behavior noted during the prenatal visits

2. The nurse monitoring a patient who is experiencing a miscarriage episode

must consider which of the following facts?

A. Miscarriages occurring before the sixth week of pregnancy often result in severe bleeding and hypovolemia.

B. A D&C can be performed to prevent a threatened miscarriage from advancing to an imminent miscarriage.

C. A missed miscarriage will result in no expulsion of blood or fetal material until the fetus actually dies.

D. Incomplete miscarriages present a greater potential for hemorrhage than do complete miscarriages.

3. If an Rh-negative woman experiences an miscarriage during her first pregnancy, she should be instructed to do which of the following?

A. Adopt children, since future pregnancies will result in future miscarriages.

B. Avoid pregnancy for the next year to permit a decrease in Rh antigens.

C. Consume high doses of vitamin D and vitamin K to prevent anemia.

D. Receive RhO immune globulin to prevent the buildup of antibodies.

4. When assessing a woman who is suspected of having an ectopic pregnancy, the nurse would report which of the following as a risk factor?

A. A history of using intrauterine devices for birth control

B. Nausea and vomiting during early pregnancy

C. A soft, nontender abdomen with active bowel sounds

D. Absence of vaginal bleeding or menstrual flow

5. Which of the following findings might be noted in a patient with a hydatidiform mole?

A. False-negative blood test results for pregnancy

B. Fetal heart tones that are louder and faster than normal

C. Marked (extreme) nausea and vomiting noted in early pregnancy

D. Uterine growth occurring more slowly than in normal pregnancy

6. Which of the following nursing diagnoses may be indicated for a patient diagnosed and treated for hydatidiform mole?

A. Altered nutrition, more than body requirements related to increased appetite

B. Fluid overload related to polycythemia due to drug therapy

C. Impaired adjustment related to incomplete grieving of lost pregnancy

D. Ineffective family coping related to poor bonding with newborn

7. Dee Ball is admitted with placenta previa with 75% coverage of the cervical os. The fetus is at 35 weeks' gestation. Which of the following nursing measures should be implemented?

A. Encourage Ms. Ball to lie on her back as much as possible.

B. Instruct Ms. Ball to use a tampon to halt the vaginal bleeding.

C. Obtain oxygen equipment to keep on standby in case the fetal heart sounds indicate fetal distress.

D. Teach Ms. Ball the importance of limiting stair-climbing to one flight during the later stages of pregnancy.

8. To determine if a patient with abruptio placentae is developing disseminated intravascular coagulation, the nurse should do which of the following?

   A. Administer heparin and perform a finger stick clotting test.

   B. Draw 5 mL of blood and monitor for clot formation.

   C. Monitor lab work for elevated levels of fibrinogen.

   D. Push fluids, then monitor for an elevated hemoglobin level.

9. Which of the following would be cause for concern if it were noted during a prenatal assessment in the third trimester?

   A. Frequent painless urination

   B. Fetal movement after eating

   C. Back pain and problems finding a comfortable sleeping position

   D. An additional, severe pain occurring with each contraction

10. Postmature pregnancy is dangerous to the fetus in which of the following ways?

    A. The fetus will suffer from decreased blood perfusion.

    B. Fetal inhalation results in aspiration of amniotic fluid.

    C. Hydramnios leading to decreased fetal circulation will occur.

    D. Microcephaly may result in increased biparietal diameter.

11. Which of the following is true about Rh incompatibility?

    A. If the mother is Rh negative and the father is homozygous Rh positive, the child will have a 50% chance of being Rh negative.

    B. If the mother is Rh negative and the father is heterozygous for the trait, 100% of the children can be expected to be Rh positive.

    C. The Rh-positive fetus inside of an Rh-negative mother is perceived as a foreign agent and stimulates the formation of antibodies.

    D. Women who are Rh negative and experience miscarriage of an Rh-positive fetus will not develop antibodies to foreign Rh antigen.

12. Which of the following observations might indicate fetal death?

    A. Failure of labor to begin before the 42nd week of gestation

    B. Reports that the fetus has been very lazy and has not moved or kicked

    C. Sonogram readings that reveal a rapid heart rate and rhythm

    D. Absence of fetal movement in the period of pregnancy prior to quickening

13. The patient going through labor who knows her child will be born dead will likely experience which of the following emotions?

    A. Relief that the pregnancy will be terminated early and she can begin to try again to have a baby

    B. Delight that she will not have to carry the heavy baby to term

    C. Grief at the loss of her infant and her inability to carry a pregnancy to term

    D. Confidence in her ability to conceive a child that will be viable

PART 2: CASE STUDY

Danielle is a 38-year-old secretary who is pregnant with her first child. She is five foot six and weighs 210 pounds. When she presents at the clinic for her seventh-month visit, the nurse notes her blood pressure is 148/92. She states she has had ankle edema for several months now but lately has noticed swelling in her face and hands.

1. What evaluation data would indicate that the nursing interventions to help control mild preeclampsia had been effective?

2. What symptoms might signal the development of pregnancy-induced hypertension? How would you teach a patient to monitor for them?

3. What nursing measures would you implement for a patient with pregnancy-induced hypertension (eclampsia)? What activities would you avoid?

■ Section Four: Inquiry and Exploration

PART 1: CRITICAL INQUIRY EXERCISES

1. Prepare a discharge teaching plan for an adolescent with preeclampsia who will be going home for the last 2 to 3 weeks of her pregnancy.

2. How might the experience of a spontaneous miscarriage in the fourth month differ for a woman who had considered termination of the pregnancy and a woman who had planned and desired the pregnancy? How might the experience be similar?

PART 2: CRITICAL EXPLORATION EXERCISES

Monitor the care of a client with preeclampsia or eclampsia. Note the nursing care provided and medications used.

Home Care
of the Pregnant Client

CHAPTER OVERVIEW

Chapter 16 discusses the usual health concerns that require home care nursing during pregnancy and the appropriate nursing actions required to identify and assist a client in the home setting. Medication therapy is reviewed and nursing implications related to the administration of medications and patient/family teaching are outlined. The use of the nursing process to plan and provide appropriate care and teaching to assist the woman with caring for herself and avoid complications is discussed.

LEARNING OBJECTIVES

After mastering the contents of this chapter, you should be able to:

1. Describe common health concerns requiring home care during pregnancy.

2. Assess the pregnant woman receiving home care.

3. Formulate nursing diagnoses related to care of the pregnant client at home.

4. Identify expected outcomes for the woman and family requiring home care.

5. Plan nursing care appropriate to meet the needs of the pregnant home care client.

6. Implement nursing care to meet the needs of the pregnant home care client.

7. Evaluate outcomes for effectiveness and achievement of a satisfying experience for the woman and her family.

8. Identify National Health Goals related to home care during pregnancy that nurses can be instrumental in helping the nation to achieve.

9. Identify areas of home care nursing that could benefit from additional nursing research or application of evidence-based practice.

10. Use critical thinking to analyze how home care influences family functioning, and develop ways to make nursing care more family-centered.

11. Integrate knowledge of home care with nursing process to achieve quality maternal and child health nursing care.

KEY TERMS

home care
perinatal home care
skilled nursing care

■ Section One:
Identification of Key Terms and Concepts

Match the terms in Part A with a definition or related statement from Part B. Place the letter corresponding to the answer in the space provided. (Letters may be used only once; some letters may not be used.)

PART A

1. _____ Total parenteral nutrition

2. _____ Perinatal home care

3. _____ Post-visit planning

4. _____ Skilled home care

PART B

A. Provided or supervised in the home by a home or community health care agency.

B. A method of supplying complete nutrition and fluid to women with hyperemesis gravidarum

C. Infection of the fetal membranes and fluid

D. Nursing care including physician-prescribed procedures such as a dressing change

E. Documenting all information gained from the visit

■ Section Two:
Short Answer and Completion Exercises

PART 1

Complete the following fill-in-the-blank exercises.

1. The nurse should plan visits at times that are convenient for the family in order

   not to disrupt _____ _____.

2. When obtaining the health history and performing a physical exam, the nurse

   must provide _____ and _____.

3. If the home situation becomes unsafe while the nurse is visiting, the nurse

   should _____, and if the nurse and client are in danger the nurse should

   _____ the _____ _____ _____ for help.

4. A major portion of planning for home care involves reviewing with the woman

   and her family exactly what will be _____ of them and what

   _____ _____ _____ from you.

PART 2

Complete the following short answer exercises.

1. Discuss how nurses can be instrumental in helping the nation achieve National Health Goals related to prevention of preterm birth.

2. What are some major assessments the nurse should make of the client and the environment when doing home care for a woman during pregnancy?

3. Discuss how follow-up visits are planned.

■ Section Three:
Critical Thinking for Application of Essential Concepts

PART 1

Circle the letter corresponding to the appropriate answer.

1. When planning a home visit, the nurse should do which of the following?
   A. Keep his or her schedule, destination, and travel route confidential to protect client privacy.
   B. Learn the location of public phones in the neighborhood.
   C. Drop in to visit on occasion to observe the family in a realistic state.
   D. Drive straight home if he or she suspects someone is following him or her.

2. Disadvantages of home care for a pregnant woman include which of the following?
   A. Care is done in the client's home.
   B. Family members are included in the plan of care.
   C. The pregnant patient assumes a greater responsibility for monitoring her condition.
   D. Family interactions, values, and priorities are more obvious than in a health care setting.

3. Which of the following is accurate instruction the nurse might need to provide to the pregnant woman receiving home care?

   A. To promote elimination, the woman should avoid high-fiber foods.

   B. When monitoring uterine contractions, the woman should count and time the contractions for 10 minutes.

   C. The woman should alternate arms with each reading when monitoring her blood pressure.

   D. Serial fundal height measurements should be taken at the same location each time.

4. Health teaching during a home care visit

   A. provides more opportunities for one-on-one teaching than in a health care agency.

   B. would not involve childbirth education, since formal classes are available.

   C. should not intrude into home activities such as food planning.

   D. involves instructing the woman to avoid all medications unless the nurse is present.

5. Jackie's husband states he wants to help in the treatment of her preterm labor. You could instruct him to do which of the following?

   A. Walk with Jackie two times each day to help her maintain adequate exercise to prevent thrombus formation.

   B. Restrict Jackie's intake of fluids to four glasses daily to prevent pulmonary edema.

   C. Remind Jackie to monitor fetal movements once a week to watch for fetal hyperactivity.

   D. Assume responsibility for childcare and household duties to help Jackie maintain strict bed rest.

PART 2: CASE STUDY

Peg Waters, age 32, is admitted onto your unit. She is pregnant with her first child. Her husband is present and they both appear anxious because Peg has gone into labor in her 36th week of gestation.

1. Peg states, "I don't know how I'm going to manage staying at home and not working." What would the nurse's best response be, and why?

2. If Peg used intravenous medication to control premature labor, what would she need to know to manage her medication?

3. What key points would you explain to Peg to prepare her for delivery of a preterm infant if her labor is not halted?

▪ Section Four: Inquiry and Exploration

PART 1: CRITICAL INQUIRY EXERCISES

1. What key points would you address in a teaching plan for an adolescent who is on home care because she is experiencing preterm labor in her 32nd week of gestation? How would this plan differ for a 28-year-old woman? A 38-year-old woman?

2. You are supervising an unlicensed assistive personnel (UAP) in home care for a pregnant client. What are some areas you would discuss with the UAP before the first client visit?

PART 2: CRITICAL EXPLORATION EXERCISES

Accompany a home health care nurse on one or more visits to a home-bound preterm labor patient. What are the major assessments and interventions made by the nurse? What changes would you make in the patient's regimen, if any, based on your observations?

High-Risk Pregnancy: The Woman With Special Needs

CHAPTER OVERVIEW

Chapter 17 discusses nursing care related to care of the woman with special needs during pregnancy. The needs of the adolescent, the woman over age 35, the woman with a physical handicap, and the woman with a drug dependency during pregnancy are reviewed. The use of the nursing process to plan and provide appropriate teaching for the woman with special needs throughout pregnancy is explored.

LEARNING OBJECTIVES

After mastering the contents of this chapter, you should be able to:

1. Identify the characteristics of the pregnant woman who has special needs.

2. Describe the risks of pregnancy for the woman with special needs.

3. Assess the woman with special needs during pregnancy.

4. State nursing diagnoses related to pregnancy for the woman with special needs.

5. Identify expected outcomes for the pregnant woman with special needs.

6. Plan nursing care to address the special growth and development needs of the adolescent and the woman over age 40 and the specific strengths and weaknesses of the woman who is physically or cognitively challenged or drug-dependent during pregnancy.

7. Implement nursing care for a woman with special needs.

8. Evaluate outcomes to ensure that goals for care have been achieved.

9. Identify National Health Goals related to women with special needs that nurses can be instrumental in helping the nation to achieve.

10. Identify areas related to care of the woman with special needs during pregnancy that would benefit from additional nursing research or application of evidence-based practice.

11. Use critical thinking to analyze ways that nursing care of the pregnant woman with a special need can be family-centered.

12. Integrate knowledge of risks of pregnancy with age extremes, drug use, and physical or cognitive challenges with the nursing process to achieve quality maternal and child health nursing care.

KEY TERMS

autonomic dysreflexia
emancipated minor
substance dependent

■ Section One:
Identification of Key Terms and Concepts

PART 1

Match the terms in Part A with a definition or related statement from Part B. Place the letter corresponding to the answer in the space provided.

PART A

1. _____ Autonomic dysreflexia

2. _____ Substance dependent

3. _____ Cephalopelvic disproportion

4. _____ Credé maneuver

5. _____ Day history

6. _____ Egocentric phenomenon

7. _____ Nest-building behavior

8. _____ Postpartal hemorrhage

9. _____ Striae

10. _____ Varicosities

PART B

A. High risk for pregnant adolescents and women over 35 due to overdistention of the uterus or decreased uterine contractility

B. Will probably fade from the adolescent's body following pregnancy

C. Written account of nutritional practices, sleep and daily activity, use of drugs, and support/friendships of the pregnant adolescent

D. May occur due to incomplete pelvic growth; requires a cesarean birth

E. Symptoms include severe hypertension, throbbing headache, nausea, bradycardia, skin flushing, and profuse diaphoresis

F. Involves withdrawal symptoms following discontinuation of a substance.

G. Should be prevented if possible by resting daily with feet elevated and sleeping in Sims position to decrease venous congestion

H. May not be noted in women over 35 until after the amniocentesis results determine the baby is healthy

I. An adolescent belief that although she is sexually active she won't become pregnant

J. Pressing the upper anterior surface of the bladder to constrict and empty; it can be used by pregnant women with no sensation of voiding

PART 2

Indicate which nursing interventions from Part B are appropriate to address the needs of a pregnant woman with each disability listed in Part A. (Some letters will be used more than once.)

PART A

1. _____ Cerebral palsy

2. _____ Hearing impairment

3. _____ Mental retardation

4. _____ Spinal cord injury

5. _____ Visual impairment

PART B

A. Refrain from using hand motions or colors when describing objects.

B. Be sure the woman spends time with her baby while in the hospital to develop confidence in her ability to provide care.

C. Provide advance opportunities to perform the infant care tasks that will be performed at home.

D. Use written instructions when possible to ensure communication.

E. Assess the support available to assist the woman as needed.

F. Allow the mother immediate contact with the infant to relieve concerns that the child may have a disability.

G. Instruct the mother that breast-feeding is not contraindicated by her condition.

■ Section Two:
Short Answer and Completion Exercises

PART 1

Complete the following fill-in-the-blank exercises.

1. Three factors that have contributed to the inability to stop teenage pregnancies

   are _____, _____, and _____.

2. Three physical conditions that a pregnant adolescent is at high risk for

   developing are _____, _____, and _____.

3. A pregnant adolescent is regarded as an _____ _____ and can make her own

   health care decisions and sign permission for her own care.

PART 2

Complete the following short answer exercises.

1. Explain how nurses can be instrumental in helping the nation achieve the goal of reducing pregnancy among girls aged 17 and younger.

2. Discuss nursing responsibilities relative to child safety when the pregnant mother is moderately or severely retarded.

3. Discuss the reasons a pregnant woman with drug dependency might not comply with a prenatal visitation schedule or proper diet.

■ Section Three:
Critical Thinking for Application of Essential Concepts

PART 1

Circle the letter corresponding to the appropriate answer.

1. Bobby, age 14, is in her fourth month of pregnancy. To help prevent the development of anemia, the nurse would do which of the following?
   A. Tell Bobby she needs to eat a balanced meal so that she will look good and be well nourished.
   B. Instruct Bobby to report black stools, which indicate that she is bleeding internally due to iron intake.
   C. Instruct Bobby regarding the signs of labor before she completes her fifth month of pregnancy.
   D. Tell Bobby if she takes an iron supplement each day she won't have to eat foods like liver.

2. When planning a teaching strategy for the pregnant adolescent, the nurse should do which of the following?
   A. Inform the teen she should consider the needs of her baby first when eating or planning activity.
   B. Omit information related to minor pains of pregnancy to prevent the adolescent from developing hypochondria.
   C. Explain how healthy eating and exercise habits will help the teen look and feel better.
   D. Emphasize the importance of frequent urine and blood testing to ensure that she is drug-free.

3. Bonnie, 16 years old and 7 months pregnant, has been diagnosed with early symptoms of pregnancy-induced hypertension (PIH). Outcome criteria that would be appropriate for Bonnie would include which of the following?

   A. Regular performance of knee-chest exercises three times daily to strengthen her vascular system

   B. Planning how she will obtain schoolwork while resting at home until her baby is born

   C. Stating her intention to watch for pale mucous membranes and note any cravings, which are signs of PIH

   D. Verbalizing her understanding that she is ill and must remain in bed in order to get well

4. Sheila, age 41, is pregnant and has been scheduled for a serum alpha-fetoprotein level. The nurse would explain which of the following to Sheila?

   A. One purpose of the test is to determine whether a chromosomal defect is present.

   B. An amniocentesis will not provide the fetal serum specimen needed for the test.

   C. Conditions like open spinal cord cannot be diagnosed through this test.

   D. The test must be performed before the 12th week of pregnancy to prevent fetal damage.

5. Your client has a T2 spinal cord injury and is 6 months pregnant. Which of the following information should be included in pregnancy counseling for her?

   A. She will not be able to feel uterine contractions, so she will need to feel her abdomen often during the last months of pregnancy to detect the tightening that occurs with labor.

   B. She should adjust the footrests on her wheelchair so that she maintains her legs with a sharp bend at the knee to relieve the pressure on her abdomen.

   C. Pregnancy will decrease her risk for urinary tract infections since serum corticosteroid levels are increased in pregnancy.

   D. The enlarged uterus will assist her in urinating, so she will not need to use a catheter or perform the Credé method to be sure she empties her bladder.

6. Joan is in her fourth month of pregnancy and confides in the nurse that she is addicted to heroin and uses prostitution to afford her habit. The nurse should respond in which of the following ways to this information?

   A. Include tests for sexually transmitted diseases in Joan's future prenatal assessments.

   B. Prepare Joan for the high possibility that her baby will be born dead because she has taken heroin.

   C. Record on Joan's chart the need to monitor her baby for hyperbilirubinemia, a complication of heroin abuse.

   D. Tell Joan her baby is in no danger because fetal exposure to narcotics actually strengthens the liver and the lungs.

7. Which of the following factors would suggest that a woman may not be a good candidate for breastfeeding?

   A. Age 35+ years

   B. T1 spinal injury

    C. Mild mental retardation

    D. Hearing impairment

8. During the postpartal period the nurse would implement which of the following measures for the visually impaired woman to facilitate maternal-child well-being?

    A. Instruct the mother to secure a sighted assistant to help her care for her new infant after she is discharged home.

    B. Limit the time the mother has to care for her child during the first few days to prevent frustration and fatigue.

    C. Speak loudly when explaining self-care measures or infant care measures the mother must use with her baby.

    D. Stress the importance of the mother facing the infant when speaking, to establish eye-to-eye contact and develop trust.

9. Tina is a pregnant cocaine user. Which of the following, if undertaken by Tina, would indicate that a teaching plan for her had been effective?

    A. Tina plans to restrict her cocaine use to smoking a pipe during her last months of pregnancy.

    B. Tina decreases cocaine use until she has completed her pregnancy.

    C. Tina stated she will use crack instead of cocaine while she is pregnant.

    D. Tina voiced plans to seek assistance to help her stop using cocaine.

10. Which of the following is information a pregnant woman who is drug-dependent should be aware of?

    A. Her fetus may be born with drug dependency and have withdrawal symptoms.

    B. Marijuana can be used to decrease withdrawal symptoms without fetal harm.

    C. Pregnancy will temporarily take away her desire for drugs and alcohol.

    D. Regular cocaine will not cross the placental barrier, but crack cocaine will.

PART 2: CASE STUDY

Bertha, age 16, has a T1 spinal injury due to an automobile accident 2 years ago. She is 4 months pregnant and is in for her second prenatal visit.

1. What are some of the major areas you would assess to determine priorities in planning care for Bertha?

2. In what ways will Bertha's age add to the complications normally present for a pregnant woman with a spinal cord injury?

3. Discuss how teenage pregnancy can result in child abuse to the newborn.

4. What birth control measures would you suggest for Bertha during your postpartal teaching?

■ Section Four: Inquiry and Exploration

PART 1: CRITICAL INQUIRY EXERCISES

1. Prepare a teaching plan for a woman with cerebral palsy that addresses methods for maintaining an adequate rest and activity pattern.

2. Write a short essay about your feelings regarding adolescent pregnancy, women over age 40 who plan pregnancy, and women with drug addiction who become pregnant. What type of nursing care should they receive?

PART 2: CRITICAL EXPLORATION EXERCISES

Visit a prenatal clinic for women who are mentally retarded. Observe the visit of a woman at each of the levels of retardation. Note the differences and similarities in instructions given regarding activities, rest, and nutritional needs.

The Nursing Role in Caring for the Family During Labor and Birth

CHAPTER 18

The Labor Process

CHAPTER OVERVIEW

Chapter 18 provides an overview of the components and process of labor and discusses nursing care of the woman in labor. Problems and concerns that may manifest during each stage of labor are reviewed. The use of the nursing process to plan and provide care throughout the stages of labor is explored.

LEARNING OBJECTIVES

After mastering the contents of this chapter, you should be able to:

1. Describe the common theories explaining the onset and progress of labor.

2. Discuss the role of the components of labor: passenger, passage, powers, and psychological impact.

3. Assess a woman in labor, identifying the stage and progression.

4. Formulate nursing diagnoses related to the physiologic and psychological aspects.

5. Establish expected outcomes to meet the needs of the woman and her family throughout the labor process.

6. Implement nursing care for the family during labor.

7. Evaluate outcomes for achievement and effectiveness of nursing care.

8. Identify National Health Goals related to a safe labor and birth that nurses can be instrumental in helping the nation to achieve.

9. Identify areas related to labor and birth that could benefit from additional nursing research or application of evidence-based practice.

10. Use critical thinking to analyze the effectiveness of nursing care measures in meeting the needs of women in labor and their families.

11. Integrate knowledge of nursing care in labor with nursing process to achieve quality maternal and child health nursing care.

KEY TERMS

amnioinfusion	lie
attitude	lightening
breech presentation	molding
cardinal movements of labor	passage
cephalic presentation	passenger
crowning	pathologic retraction ring
dilatation	physiologic retraction ring
effacement	position
engagement	powers
episiotomy	ripening
fetal descent	station
Leopold's maneuver	transition

■ Section One: Identification of Key Terms and Concepts

PART 1

Match the terms in Column I with a definition or related statement from Part B. Place the letter corresponding to the answer in the space provided. (Letters may be used only once; some letters may not be used.)

COLUMN I

1. __D__ Attitude D

2. __K__ Crowning K

3. __H__ Amnioinfusion H

4. __B__ Effacement B

5. __A__ Engagement A

6. _____ Fontanelle C

7. __F__ Labor F

8. __E__ Molding E

9. __J__ Physiologic retraction ring J

10. _____ Power

PART B

A. Occurs when the presenting part of the fetus has settled into the pelvis at the level of the ischial spines

B. The shortening and thinning of the cervical canal

C. Membrane-covered spaces at the junction of the main suture lines

D. The degree of flexion the fetus assumes or the relation of the fetal parts to each other

E. The change in shape of the fetal skull produced by the force of uterine contractions pressing the vertex against the closed cervix

F. A series of events by which uterine contractions expel the fetus and placenta from the woman's body

G. A ridge on the inner uterine surface representing the boundary between the thick active and thinner inactive portions of the uterus

H. The addition of a sterile fluid into the pregnant uterus

I. Irregular uterine cramps, which may signal the impending onset of true labor

J. Supplied by the fundus of the uterus and supplemented by abdominal muscles; results in the expulsion of the fetus from the uterus

K. The appearance of the presenting part of the fetus at the opening of the vagina

PART 2

Match each definition or related statement in Part A with the correct fetal position in Part B. Place the letter of the answer in the space provided. (Some letters may not be used.)

PART A

1. __E__ The occiput of the fetus points to the left anterior quadrant in a vertex position.   *LOA*

2. __D__ The triangular fontanelle points toward the right anterior pelvic quadrant.

3. __F__ The fetal anus of a breech presentation is pointed toward the maternal pelvis.

4. __C__ The fetal chin is located across the pelvic midsection.

5. __A__ The fetal shoulder is located in the right lower posterior pelvic area.

PART B

a. Right scapuloposterior (RAP)   *RAP*

b. Left occipitotransverse (LOT)   *Sa*

c. Left mentotransverse (LMT)

d. Right occipitoanterior (ROA)

e. Left occipitoanterior (LOA)

f. Right sacroanterior (RSaA)

■ Section Two: Short Answer and Completion Exercises

PART 1

Complete the following fill-in-the-blank exercises.

1. During the process of labor the fetus passes from the __uterus__ through the __cervix__ and __vagina__ to the __external__ __perineum__.

2. The first division of the first stage of labor is the __preparatory__ division.

3. Three of the six signs of impending labor are __ruptured__, __show__, and __ripened cervix__
   __membranes__

4. The three integrated concepts contributing to the success of labor are whether the passenger is _____, the passage is _____, and the power or force of contraction is _____.

5. The four methods by which the fetal position, presentation, and lie are established are combined abdominal _inspection_ and _palpation_, _vag_ _exam_, auscultation of _fetal_ _heart_ _tones_, and _sonography_.

✓ 6. The softening of the cervix, which occurs in preparation for labor, is called _ripening_.

✓ 7. Following rupture of the membranes, _temp_ should be taken every 2 hours because of the possibility of infection.

8. As the fetal head moves from above to below the level of the ischial spines, the station or degree of engagement moves from _minus_ to _plus_ stations.

PART 2

Complete the following short answer exercises.

✗ 1. Discuss three of the factors that may influence the beginning of labor.

   Show = mucus plug released + capillary ln
   ruptured membranes = mucus plug
   ripened cervix = becomes butter soft

2. Discuss the role of diaphoresis in temperature regulation during labor.

   works to cool the ↑ body temp

3. Describe the resulting effect when a body part other than the vertex presents.

   ✗ - C-section, forceps
   - irreg. + weak contr'ns
   - ineffective dilation

4. Describe the process and purpose of Leopold's maneuvers.

   Leopold's maneuver systematic method of
   observation + palpation to determine fetal presentation
   and position

5. Discuss the psychological responses of a woman to labor and the nurse's role.

- fear - fatigue - anxious

- nurse - comfort,

6. Compare and contrast the changes occurring in the pulse and blood pressure of the mother with changes occurring in the fetal pulse and blood pressure during contractions.

7. Discuss the role that the father or a significant other might play in the labor experience.

8. Indicate the significance of each of the following abnormal fetal heart rate patterns: fetal tachycardia, fetal bradycardia, late deceleration, variable pattern, sinusoidal pattern.

PART 3 (p. 473)

Describe the following fetal positions that occur during the fetal descent phase:

Internal rotation

Extension - back of the neck stops beneath

External rotation

Expulsion

■ Section Three:
Critical Thinking for Application of Essential Concepts

PART 1

Circle the letter corresponding to the appropriate answer.

1. Bobby has been experiencing regular, coordinated contractions with cervical dilation moving from 4 cm to 6 cm in the last half-hour, and her membranes are still intact. Bobby is in which of the following stages of labor?

    A. Latent phase of the second stage of labor

    B. Active phase of the first stage of labor

    C. Placental stage or the third stage of labor

    D. Predelivery stage or the prelabor stage of labor

2. When planning comfort measures to help the woman in active labor tolerate her pain, the nurse must consider which of the following?

    A. Early labor contractions are usually regular, coordinated, and very painful.

    B. If women are properly prepared, they will require no medication to manage their pain.

    C. Pain medication given during the latent phase of labor is not likely to impair contractions.

    D. The active phase of labor can be a time of true discomfort and high anxiety.

3. Bonnie, 14 years of age, is in labor and expresses the following concern: "The doctor said the baby might not be able to be vaginally delivered because of some disproportion. What is wrong with my baby?" The nurse should discuss which of the following with Bonnie?

    A. The cause of pelvic disproportion due to the poor eating habits exhibited by adolescents during pregnancy

    B. Methods of stretching cervical musculature through exercise to facilitate vaginal delivery

    C. The fact that pelvic disproportion is usually caused by a problem with the size of the pelvis, not the size of the fetus

    D. The complications that can result from the fetus being pushed against a small or undilated pelvic opening

4. Sheila is in her first stage of labor and the nurse notices a distinct abdominal indentation that she recognizes as a retraction ring. The nurse should respond to these findings by doing which of the following?

    A. Inform Sheila that this indentation is normal, to decrease her anxiety.

    B. Instruct Sheila to lie on her right side to prevent pressure on her abdomen.

    C. Recognize this as an indication that labor is almost complete.

    D. Report this danger sign to the physician immediately.

5. Frances is admitted in active labor. The nurse locates fetal heart sounds in the upper left quadrant of her abdomen. The nurse would recognize which of the following?

    A. Frances will probably deliver very quickly and without problems.

    B. This indicates Frances will probably have a breech delivery.

C. The fetus is in the most common anterior fetal position.

D. This position is referred to as being left anteriopelvic.

6. While interviewing a woman in labor, the nurse would address which of the following?

   A. Whether the pregnancy was planned

   B. The use of drugs or medications during pregnancy

   C. Maternal concerns regarding fetal health

   D. All of the above

7. When timing the length of a contraction, the nurse would do which of the following?

   A. Ask the woman when the beginning of the contraction is felt, then time the interval from this point until the woman states the contraction has subsided.

   B. Gently palpate the abdomen for the beginning of the tightening of the uterus; time the interval from this point until the uterine tightening subsides.

   C. Lightly touch the abdomen and time the interval from the beginning of the uterine tensing to the beginning of the next tensing.

   D. Note the upward slopes of the contraction on the monitor graph and measure from one upward slope to the next upward slope.

8. Which of the following is very important when performing fetal monitoring?

   A. Informing the mother and significant others that the fetal heart rate will vary during the labor process

   B. Instructing the mother that she must lie supine to obtain the most accurate readings of fetal status

   C. Keeping the monitor strap on the woman's abdomen tightly and securely fitted despite maternal discomfort

   D. Maintaining a continuous watch on the monitor, since it is the primary source of data on maternal-fetal status

9. Internal monitoring has which of the following characteristics?

   A. Little restriction on maternal ambulation

   B. Can be applied before rupture of the membranes

   C. A clearer printout of the fetal heart rate

   D. Cannot be initiated if the fetal head is engaged

10. Fetal distress is suspected if which of the following diagnostic results is obtained?

    A. Fetal heart rate acceleration occurring with scalp stimulation

    B. Early decelerations indicated on the fetal heart monitor

    C. Serial blood specimen readings reveal pH levels of 7.10 to 7.15

    D. Fetus is positioned in the left occipitoanterior area

11. If variable deceleration is noted on the fetal heart monitor, the nurse should do which of the following?

    A. Limit oral and intravenous fluids to decrease maternal fluid volume and decrease circulatory overload.

    B. Prepare a needle and large syringe so the physician can remove the excess amniotic fluid causing the problem.

    C. Remove oxygen, if present, and instruct the mother to breathe slowly, since this is a sign of hyperventilation.

    D. Turn the mother to a different position to relieve pressure on the umbilical cord and restore circulation.

12. If a woman will be placing her baby up for adoption, which of the following nursing measures should be implemented during labor?

    A. Avoid discussing the baby during the historical assessment to minimize the woman's anxiety.

    B. Support the woman as needed by accepting the decisions she makes regarding holding the baby.

    C. Protect the woman from visitors and family members who might try to change her mind.

    D. Take the baby away as soon as possible after birth to prevent bonding from occurring.

13. After the third stage of labor the nurse may have which of the following responsibilities?

    A. Administration of intramuscular oxytocin to facilitate uterine contractility

    B. Monitoring for blood loss greater than 60 cc, which would indicate gross hemorrhage

    C. Noting if the placenta makes a Schultze presentation, which is a sign of gross complications

    D. Pushing down on the relaxed uterus to aid in the removal of the placenta

14. Immediately after episiotomy repair, the nurse would do which of the following?

    A. Cleanse the woman's anal area, then perineum and vulva, to remove any fecal incontinence or vaginal secretions.

    B. Monitor the woman for shaking and complaints of chill sensations, which may indicate an adverse reaction to medications.

    C. Palpate the uterine fundus for size, consistency, and position, and take vital signs to obtain baseline data.

    D. Remove all coverings except a clean, light hospital gown to prevent the development of postpartal fever.

15. Which of the following outcome criteria would be appropriate for the woman in labor without a support person?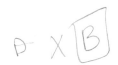

    A. Reuniting with her child's father before labor is complete

    B. Verbalizing that she felt supported during the labor process

    C. Indicating that she was comfortable going through labor alone

    D. Stating the labor process was a smooth, rewarding experience

16. Which of the following signs could indicate maternal distress?
    A. Heart rate of 90 to 100 beats per minute during labor
    B. Less frequent, less intense uterine contractions
    C. Reports of feeling the need to have a bowel movement
    D. Uterine relaxation between 60-second contractions

17. Which of the following is true about vaginal births following cesarean birth?
    A. Instructions regarding the labor process are not needed.
    B. Many women will respond as if this is their first pregnancy.
    C. Recent studies have shown this to be a dangerous practice.
    D. Women usually prefer cesarean birth to vaginal delivery.

PART 2: CASE STUDY

Effie is a 21-year-old primipara who has completed natural childbirth classes with her coach, her husband. She is admitted at noon to the birthing room after 3 hours of active labor at home. She is dilated 3 cm and 80% effaced. Her sister is with her, and she is concerned about causing her husband to miss time at work needlessly early. He is a low-paid hourly worker, and they are a one-income family.

1. What would you explain to Effie about the progression of her labor, and how would you advise her regarding contacting her husband?

2. How could you support Effie, or teach the family to support Effie, if her husband was not present during the second state of her labor?

3. If labor failed to progress, what additional types of support might Effie need? How might these supports differ for a woman who had a prior delivery by cesarean birth?

4. How would your support for Effie differ if she were a woman who had previously had a difficult delivery?

■ Section Four:
Inquiry and Exploration

PART 1: CRITICAL INQUIRY EXERCISES

1. Prepare a teaching plan for a woman in labor that addresses methods for maintaining a maximum state of comfort during the first and second stages of labor.

2. Briefly explain how you would support a woman who has decided to put her baby up for adoption through the labor process. How would your support measures differ, if at all, for an adolescent girl?

PART 2: CRITICAL EXPLORATION EXERCISES

Chart the progression of a woman in the active phases of labor on commercial graph forms or using square-ruled graph paper. Note if the progression appears normal or abnormal by comparison with the chart presented in your text.

Providing Comfort During Labor and Birth

CHAPTER OVERVIEW

Chapter 19 provides an overview of the physiology and perception of pain during labor and principles of pain management, including pharmacologic methods and support of the woman's chosen technique for relaxation and prepared childbirth. The use of the nursing process to plan and provide comfort for the woman throughout labor and delivery is explored.

LEARNING OBJECTIVES

After mastering the contents of this chapter, you should be able to:

1. Describe the physiologic basis of contractions during labor and birth and related theories of pain relief.

2. Identify complementary and alternative therapies that may be used to promote a woman's comfort during labor and birth.

3. Discuss the pharmacologic agents commonly used to provide analgesia and anesthesia.

4. Assess the degree and type of discomfort a woman is experiencing, including her ability to cope with it effectively during labor and birth.

5. Formulate nursing diagnoses related to the effect of pain during labor and birth.

6. Establish expected outcomes to meet the needs of the woman experiencing discomfort during labor and birth.

7. Plan nursing interventions to promote comfort during labor and birth.

8. Implement common complementary and pharmacologic measures for pain relief during labor and birth.

9. Evaluate outcomes for effectiveness of nursing care and achievement of a satisfying labor experience for the woman and her family.

10. Identify National Health Goals related to anesthesia and childbirth that nurses can be instrumental in helping the nation achieve.

11. Identify areas related to promoting comfort during labor that could benefit from additional nursing research or application of evidence-based practice.

12. Use critical thinking to analyze ways to maintain family-centered care when analgesia and anesthesia are used in childbirth.

13. Integrate knowledge of pain relief measures during labor and birth using the nursing process to achieve quality maternal and child nursing care.

KEY TERMS

analgesia	pain
anesthesia	pressure anesthesia
doula	pudendal nerve block
endorphin	transcutaneous electrical nerve stimulation (TENS)
epidural anesthesia	

■ Section One:
Identification of Key Terms and Concepts

Match the terms in Part A with a definition or related statement from Part B. Place the letter corresponding to the answer in the space provided. (Letters may be used only once; some letters may not be used.)

PART A

1. __I__ Aspiration

2. __C__ Endorphin

3. __G__ Spinal anesthesia

4. __J__ General anesthesia

5. __E__ Pain

6. __B__ Meperidine

7. __A__ Pudendal nerve block

8. __D__ Regional anesthesia

9. __F__ Transcutaneous electrical nerve stimulation (TENS)

PART B

A. Injection of anesthetic at the level of the ischial spine; allows for low forceps delivery and episiotomy repair

B. A synthetic narcotic with sedative and antispasmodic action

C. Opiate-like substance produced naturally by the body to reduce pain

D. Results in minimal fetal effects compared with systemic anesthetics; leaves the uterus capable of optimal postpartal contraction

E. A subjective symptom; any sensation of discomfort

F. Blocks afferent fibers, preventing pain from traveling to the spinal cord synapses from the uterus; also effective with extreme back pain

G. A local anesthetic agent injected into the third lumbar space

H. Pharmacologic pain management that causes partial or complete loss of sensation

I. Inhalation of vomitus that may cause occlusion of the airway

J. Not a preferred method of pain control in childbirth; requires maternal intubation and increases the risk of aspiration

K. Introduction of an anesthetic agent into the dura mater

■ Section Two:
Short Answer and Completion Exercises

PART 1

Complete the following fill-in-the-blank exercises.

1. When using pain control drugs during labor and delivery, the risks of fetal
   bradycardia and maternal hypotension must be weighed against the alternative
   risk to the mother, which would be _enduring_ _a_ _painful_
   labor.

2. Nurses can help the nation meet the goals of reducing maternal and fetal
   deaths related to analgesia and anesthesia administered during labor and birth
   by _____, _____, and _____.

3. During uterine contractions of labor, the two major sources of pain are
   _____ and _____.

4. During the first stage of labor, pain relief must either be _systemic_ or block
   the synapse sites at spinal column level _T₁₀_ through _L₁_.

5. Effective medication for pain management during labor must not only relieve
   the woman's pain, but must also _relax_ the woman, have minimal
   systemic effects, and have minimal effects on uterine _contraction_ her
   pushing _effort_, and the fetus.

PART 2

Complete the following short answer exercises.

1. Discuss the significance of informing a woman of the use of drugs and the
   ultimate effect of the various pain relief measures before the choice of a pain
   relief medication.

2. Explain how knowledge regarding the labor and delivery process might have
   an impact on the pain experienced during labor.

3. Discuss the importance of timing in the administration of pain relief medications during labor.

4. Discuss the role that a significant other might play in facilitating pain relief during the labor experience.

PART 3

Indicate the likelihood of fetal effect from the drug type listed (yes or no).

1. _____ Molecular weight above 1,000

2. _____ Molecular weight below 600

3. _____ Drugs that strongly bind to protein

4. _____ Fat-soluble drugs

5. _____ Drugs administered to a woman with a premature fetus

6. _____ Drugs that cause systemic maternal hypotension

■ Section Three:
Critical Thinking for Application of Essential Concepts

PART 1

Circle the letter corresponding to the appropriate answer.

1. Barbara, a primipara, has been experiencing regular contractions with cervical dilation at 2 cm. Barbara could use which of the following pain relief measures safely?
   A. Acetylsalicylic acid
   B. Breathing exercises
   C. Narcotic analgesic
   D. Pressure anesthesia

2. When planning comfort measures to help the woman in active labor tolerate her pain, the nurse must consider which of the following?
   A. Early labor contractions are usually regular, coordinated, and very painful.
   B. If women are properly prepared, they are more likely to require less medication to manage their pain.

CHAPTER 19 ■ **Providing Comfort During Labor and Birth** **125**

C. Pain medication given during the latent phase of labor is not likely to impair contractions.

D. The acceleration phase of labor represents a time of minimum pain and discomfort.

3. Which of the following actions should the nurse take when administering Demerol (meperidine) to a woman in labor?

A. Administer a dose of Narcan with the medication to boost the antianxiety effects.

B. Inject the medication into the woman's subcutaneous tissue.

C. Monitor the infant for sedation for 3 to 4 hours after the drug is administered.

D. Reassure the woman that this drug does not cross the placenta.

4. The nurse could feel most comfortable with the administration of which of the following medications to a woman with known heart or pulmonary disease?

A. An epidural block

B. General anesthesia

C. Narcotic analgesics

D. Patient-controlled analgesia

5. Which of the following measures could a nurse take to facilitate comfort in the labor process?

A. Apply a sanitary pad to decrease discomfort from vaginal secretions.

B. If membranes are ruptured and the fetus is not engaged, encourage ambulation around the room.

C. Smooth the wrinkles from bed linen and remove sticky bedclothes.

D. Tell the woman to remain as still as possible throughout the labor process to decrease stimulation.

PART 2: CASE STUDY

Alice and Mike are in the birthing room performing breathing exercises during her third hour of true labor. This is their first pregnancy and birth. Alice is dilated 4 cm. Mike appears nervous but is enthusiastic and caring in his coaching.

1. What impact could Mike's nervousness have on Alice and the progress of her labor? What nursing actions would be indicated to address his nervousness?

2. Alice has asked about the risks of using a narcotic analgesic to relieve her pain now. What information would you give her regarding the benefits and disadvantages of analgesic agents at this stage in her labor?

3. What information would you give Alice and Mike about pain control during the second and third phases of labor?

■ Section Four: Inquiry and Exploration

PART 1: CRITICAL INQUIRY EXERCISES

1. Prepare a pain management plan for a woman in labor that includes two nonpharmacologic pain relief measures and two medical pain relief methods, with nursing implications for monitoring and prevention of drug-related complications.

2. Prepare a checklist of the priority assessments and related nursing actions for managing pain in each stage of labor.

PART 2: CRITICAL EXPLORATION EXERCISES

Monitor a woman through the entire labor process. Note the methods used by the woman and the health care team to maintain a maximum state of comfort during the first and second stages of labor.

CHAPTER 20

Cesarean Birth

CHAPTER OVERVIEW

Interruptions in the predictable laboring process and the mechanics of delivery may require a woman to be prepared to deliver her infant by cesarean birth. This chapter reviews both scheduled and emergency cesarean births and examines the pre- and postoperative principles of nursing for the client experiencing a cesarean surgery. Reasons for cesarean birth, the surgical procedure, and physiological and psychological responses of the woman are discussed.

LEARNING OBJECTIVES

After mastering the contents of this chapter, you should be able to:

1. Describe the indications for cesarean birth.

2. Assess a woman scheduled for cesarean birth for effective preoperative, intraoperative, and postoperative needs.

3. Formulate nursing diagnoses related to cesarean birth.

4. Establish outcomes that meet the needs of a woman requiring a cesarean birth.

5. Plan appropriate nursing care to ensure family-centered care.

6. Implement common preoperative and postoperative care measures for cesarean birth.

7. Evaluate outcomes for achievement and effectiveness of nursing care.

8. Identify National Health Goals related to cesarean birth that nurses can be instrumental in helping the nation to achieve.

9. Identify areas related to cesarean birth that could benefit from additional nursing research or application of evidence-based practice.

10. Use critical thinking to analyze common complications of cesarean birth to develop preventive strategies.

11. Integrate knowledge of cesarean birth with the nursing process to achieve quality maternal and child health nursing care.

KEY TERMS

cesarean birth
classic cesarean incision
dehiscence
low segment incision
retractors

■ Section One: Identification of Key Terms and Concepts

PART 1

Match the terms in Part A with a definition or related statement from Part B. Place the letter corresponding to the answer in the space provided.

PART A

1. _B_ Transcutaneous electrical nerve stimulation (TENS)
2. _C_ Patient-controlled analgesia (PCA)
3. _D_ Stress response
4. _A_ Epidural analgesia

4/4

PART B

A. May result in intense itching and nausea and vomiting
B. Applying electrodes to the surface of the skin to effectively control pain by blocking the ability of the cerebral cortex to interpret the incoming sensation
C. Self-administration of intravenous narcotic analgesia
D. Results in the release of epinephrine and norepinephrine from the adrenal gland medulla

PART 2

Indicate if the following statements are true or false by placing a "T" or "F" in the space provided.

1. _T_ Obesity may predispose a surgical client's skin line repair to dehiscence.
2. _F_ Unlike the cesarean birth client who has received general anesthesia, the cesarean birth client who has received an epidural is not at risk for intestinal paralysis.
X 3. _T_ The woman who was anesthetized by an epidural procedure is limited to a supine position immediately after surgery.
5. _F_ Lochia should not be visible for assessment if the woman has a cesarean birth.

■ Section Two: Short Answer and Completion Exercises

Complete the following short answer exercises.

1. During a vaginal delivery a woman loses ___300___ to ___500___ mL of blood as compared to a cesarean birth where she loses ___500___ to ___1000___ mL.

2. What are the basic physiological and psychological factors that may predispose a client who has experienced a cesarean procedure to a complicated surgical outcome?

3. Why is it a good nursing action to include the expectant woman's support person when giving anticipatory guidance?

4. Why is a sonogram useful to the physician prior to making the incision for a cesarean procedure?

5. Explain why it is of utmost importance that the surgical client be assessed for urinary output following surgery.

6. Identify and discuss three potential maladaptations that may occur in a woman following a cesarean birth procedure if her pain is not controlled.

    1) interference ē bonding   2) Thrombophlebitis   3) Pneumonia

7. Identify and discuss two supportive pain control devices that can be used to assist the postpartal surgical client. Explain the essential components of these devices.

▪ Section Three:
Critical Thinking for Application of Essential Concepts

PART 1

Circle the letter corresponding to the appropriate answer.

1. Mrs. Jordan has been admitted on the maternity ward the day prior to a scheduled cesarean birth. Mrs. Jordan is unable to deliver vaginally due to cephalopelvic disproportion. The nurse instructs Mrs. Jordan on deep breathing exercises as part of the preoperative teaching plan. The rationale for this exercise is to

    A. promote involution on a traumatized uterus.

    B. prevent stasis of mucus in the lungs.

    C. prevent pulmonary edema.

    D. stimulate the diaphragm to contract.

     B

2. The nurse administers ranitidine (Zantac) prior to surgery to

    A. neutralize gastric secretions.

    B. promote uterine contractions.

    C. delay uterine contractions.

    D. decrease gastric secretions.

    D

3. The surgeon plans to perform a low segment incision rather than a classic cesarean. The low cervical incision is more advantageous because

   A. it is made horizontally and high on the woman's abdomen.

   B. the procedure is faster since the incision is made through the abdomen and uterus at the same time.

   C. the likelihood of a postpartal uterine infection is decreased.

   D. the procedure is made with a vertical incision to decrease the chances of reopening.

   C

4. As the nurse cares for Mrs. Jordan after her cesarean section, she will implement measures to prevent peritonitis. A positive sign that this illness is present would be a(n)

   A. guarded abdomen.

   B. elevated temperature.

   C. excessive lochia discharge.

   D. episode of painful involuntary retractions.

5. If oxytocin is ordered as a medical regimen postoperatively for the client who has had a cesarean birth, the most important nursing intervention would be to

   A. monitor the blood pressure.

   B. monitor the increased lochia discharge.

   C. prevent infection at the incision site.

   D. implement measures to promote comfort.

   A

PART 2: CASE STUDY

Lorraine Murphy has delivered her first child under general anesthesia by the cesarean method. The nurse will need to monitor her closely for postpartal and postsurgical complications.

1. What position should Ms. Murphy be placed in when she is brought to the recovery room? Specify how you may help the patient maintain this position.

2. Explain why Ms. Murphy would be in jeopardy for an imbalance of fluid and electrolytes. What important vital signs may alert you to this problem? What drug might be ordered by the physician to ensure uterine contractions?

3. Ms. Murphy has begun to wake up; her words are barely audible, but she manages to ask you for something to drink. How would you respond?

■ Section Four: Inquiry and Exploration

PART 1: CRITICAL INQUIRY EXERCISES

1. Formulate a nursing care plan that will focus on alleviating fears for the client and family awaiting a cesarean delivery.

2. Compare the pre- and postoperative nursing care needed for the client who delivers vaginally with the client who has undergone a cesarean section delivery.

PART 2: CRITICAL EXPLORATION EXERCISES

Formulate a teaching plan for a pregnant woman whom you will care for when assigned to the women's health unit. The plan should indicate that this patient has been scheduled for a preplanned surgical procedure. Identify those teaching advantages from your text that you propose will enable the nurse to prepare the patient more efficiently due to the nature of the birthing method. After you have been assigned to the patient on the floor, compare and contrast the teaching points that you selected from your text with those listed in the teaching care plan on the patient's chart.

The Woman Who Develops a Complication During Labor and Birth

CHAPTER OVERVIEW

Chapter 21 describes and summarizes the more common complications that occur during labor and birth. Women who are most at risk are discussed. The chapter also explores the planning and implementation of care for high-risk women in labor. Common treatments are explained and illustrated. Nursing diagnoses and related intervention skills are emphasized.

LEARNING OBJECTIVES

After mastering the contents of this chapter, you should be able to:

1. Define the terms dystocia and dysfunctional labor

2. Describe the common deviations in the power (force of labor), the passage, or passenger that can cause dystocia or dysfunctional labor.

3. Assess the woman in labor and during birth for deviations from the normal labor process.

4. Formulate nursing diagnoses related to deviations from the normal labor process.

5. Identify appropriate outcomes associated with deviations in normal labor and birth and resultant complications.

6. Plan nursing interventions that will help the family meet established outcomes.

7. Implement care related to potential complications in labor or birth.

8. Evaluate outcomes for achievement and effectiveness of care.

9. Identify National Health Goals related to complications of labor that nurses could be instrumental in helping the nation achieve.

10. Identify areas related to complications of labor that could benefit from additional nursing research or application of evidence-based practice.

11. Use critical thinking to analyze ways to maintain family-centered nursing care when deviations from the normal in labor and birth occur.

12. Integrate the knowledge of deviations from normal in labor and birth with nursing process to achieve quality maternal and child health nursing care.

KEY TERMS

amniotic fluid embolism
augmentation of labor
battledore placenta
cephalopelvic disproportion
constriction ring
dysfunctional labor
dystocia
external cephalic version
forceps birth
hypertonic uterine contractions
hypotonic uterine contractions

induction of labor
oxytocin
pathologic retraction ring
placenta accreta
placenta circumvallata
placenta marginata
placenta succenturiata
precipitate labor
umbilical cord prolapse
uterine inversion
vacuum extraction

■ Section One:
Identification of Key Terms and Concepts

PART 1

Match the terms in Part A with a definition or related statement from Part B. Place the letter corresponding to the answer in the space provided.

PART A

1. _____ Cephalopelvic disproportion

2. _____ Cervical ripening

3. _____ Oxytocin

4. _____ Dystocia

5. _____ McRobert's maneuver

6. _____ Pathologic retraction ring

7. _____ Vacuum extraction

8. _____ Uterine inversion

9. _____ Piper forceps

10. _____ External cephalic version

PART B

A. Has an advantage over forceps births

B. Used to deliver the head in a breech presentation

C. Ridge across abdomen that signals possible uterine rupture

D. Uterus turns inside out

E. Drug used to induce or augment labor

F. Gentle external pressure used to rotate the position of the fetus

G. Sharply flexing the woman's thighs onto the abdomen

H. Fetal head too large for passage; small pelvis

I. Change in consistency from firm to soft

J. Sluggishness of contractions or force of labor

PART 2

Indicate whether the following dysfunctions occur in the first (A) or second (B) stage of labor by placing an "A" or "B" in the space provided.

1. _____ Protracted active phase

2. _____ Prolonged deceleration phase

3. _____ Arrest of descent

4. _____ Prolonged descent

5. _____ Secondary arrest of dilation

6. _____ Prolonged latent phase

7. _____ Failure to descend

■ Section Two:
Short Answer and Completion Exercises

PART 1

Complete the following fill-in-the-blank exercises.

1. Management of a prolapsed cord is aimed toward relieving _____
   _____ _____ _____ , which will relieve _____
   _____ and fetal _____.

2. Immediate management of umbilical cord prolapse is to place the patient in a
   _____-_____ position or _____ position.

3. _____ _____ or _____ labor are terms used to describe sluggish
   contractions.

4. _____ _____ is the surgical treatment of choice for many types of abnormal
   labor.

5. _____ _____ _____ _____ is a warning sign of severe
   dysfunctional labor and may signal an impending _____ of the
   uterus.

6. Umbilical cords that have only two vessels are associated with congenital
   _____ and _____ anomalies.

PART 2

Complete the following exercises.

1. List and define the three main components of labor.

   _____   _____

   _____

2. Name the chief assessment measures used to detect deviations from normal labor and birth.

3. List three types of abnormal uterine contractions.

   _____   _____

   _____

4. Name the dysfunctional labor phases of the primary state of labor.

5. Name three common health problems associated with multiple gestation deliveries.

   _____   _____

   _____

6. List two dangers of a breech delivery.

   _____   _____

7. List four types of abnormal presentation.

   _____   _____

   _____   _____

8. Describe two nontherapeutic effects of oxytocin.

   _____   _____

9. Name three indications for a forceps delivery.

   _____   _____

   _____

10. List the four types of breech presentation.

    _____   _____

    _____   _____

11. List six conditions that are a high risk for a prolapsed cord.

_____   _____

_____   _____

_____   _____

12. Name six conditions that may place the patient at high risk for uterine rupture during the birthing process.

_____   _____

_____   _____

_____   _____

■ Section Three:
Critical Thinking for Application of Essential Concepts

PART 1

Circle the letter corresponding to the appropriate answer.

1. Labor may be induced in which of the following women? A woman with:
   A. a fetus in transverse lie.
   B. presenting part engaged.
   C. a premature fetus.
   D. cephalopelvic disproportion.

2. Standard care plans for a woman in normal active labor include
   A. explanation of all procedures being performed.
   B. assessment to determine that the resting tone of the uterus is maintained above 15 mm Hg.
   C. use of sedation, whenever requested.
   D. preparing for administration of Pitocin (oxytocin) and use of high forceps.

3. A multiparous woman arrived 2 hours ago in active labor with 4 cm of cervical dilation. Now she states that she has a strong urge to push. Which answer most likely describes what is occurring?
   A. She may have cephalopelvic disproportion.
   B. She may need an analgesic or sedation.
   C. She is having a precipitous delivery.
   D. She is having a breech birth.

4. The nurse would prepare for treatment of amniotic fluid embolism with which of the following clients? The client:
   A. reporting sudden severe chest pain and dyspnea
   B. demonstrating hypotonic contractions and poor force of labor
   C. experiencing back pain when ambulating or lying in bed
   D. receiving a tocolytic to treat precipitate labor

5. To assess a laboring client for ineffective uterine force the nurse would:

   A. check the electrolyte panel for the level of carbon dioxide.

   B. obtain a specimen of amniotic fluid and assess for glucose.

   C. calculate Montevideo units through electronic monitoring.

   D. watch the client for elevated respiratory rates during contractions.

6. A woman with a fetus in occipitoposterior position would commonly demonstrate which of the following?

   A. precipitate labor

   B. acute chest pain

   C. increased energy levels.

   D. intense back pressure

PART 2: CASE STUDY

Mrs. Price, age 36, is in premature labor, expecting twins. She is at 36 weeks' gestation, and one of the twins is a breech presentation. This is Mrs. Price's second multiple birth. Her previous delivery of twins resulted in the death of twin A; twin B survived and was later diagnosed with cerebral palsy.

1. What concerns might Mr. and Mrs. Price voice about the impending cesarean section?

2. How should the nurse prepare to respond to their questions and their anxiety?

3. While preparing Mrs. Price for the cesarean section, what changes and vital signs might you assess that would indicate the development of additional problems or complications for Mrs. Price?

4. Explain why Mrs. Price is at risk for an alteration in fluid and electrolyte balance.

■ Section Four:
Inquiry and Exploration

PART 1: CRITICAL INQUIRY EXERCISES

1. Choose a potential health problem as a complication of labor and write a care plan for this high-risk patient.

2. Formulate a nursing care plan for a woman who is pregnant with her first child and is in prolonged labor.

PART 2: CRITICAL EXPLORATION EXERCISES

Arrange to visit the labor and delivery care areas in your hospital. Seek assistance from the staff to accompany and monitor a patient who would need surgery after her labor has failed to progress.

The Nursing Role in Caring for the Family During the Postpartal Period

Nursing Care of the Postpartal Woman and Family

CHAPTER OVERVIEW

Chapter 22 presents an overview of the physiologic and psychological care of the postpartal woman and family. The physiologic changes that occur after childbirth and the emotional effects of childbirth on the entire postpartal family are discussed. The use of the nursing process to plan and provide care for the postpartal family is explored.

LEARNING OBJECTIVES

After mastering the contents of this chapter, you should be able to:

1. Describe the psychological and physiologic changes that occur in the postpartal woman.

2. Use the nursing process to determine and address nursing diagnoses related to the physiologic and psychological changes experienced by the postpartal woman and her family during the postpartal period.

3. Identify National Health Goals related to the postpartal period that nurses can be instrumental in helping the nation achieve.

4. Use critical thinking to analyze ways that postpartal nursing care can be more family-centered.

5. Synthesize knowledge of the physiologic and psychological changes of the postpartal period using the nursing process to achieve quality maternal and child health nursing care.

KEY TERMS

afterpains
diastasis recti
en face position
engorgement
engrossment
Homans' sign
involution
letting-go phase

lochia alba
lochia rubra
lochia serosa
primary encouragement
sitz bath
taking-hold phase
taking-in phase
uterine atony

■ Section One: Identification of Key Terms and Concepts

PART 1

Match the terms in Part A with a definition or related statement from Part B. Place the letter corresponding to the answer in the space provided.

PART A

1. _____ Uterine tone assessment

2. _____ Empty bladder

3. _____ Primary engorgement

4. _____ Hydronephrosis

5. _____ 2,200 to 2,300 kcal, high-protein diet

6. _____ Early ambulating

7. _____ Sitz bath

8. _____ Immediate maternal-child contact

9. _____ Oral contraception

10. _____ Follow-up examination visit

PART B

A. Needed to promote tissue healing

B. Decreased opportunity for infection and promotes comfort

C. Tension feeling of breast on day 3 or 4 postpartum

D. Increased size of ureters during pregnancy

E. Can be resumed 2 to 3 weeks postpartum

F. Detects potential for postpartum hemorrhage

G. Occurs 4 to 6 weeks after delivery

H. Decreases constipation and urinary retention

I. Prevents displacement of the uterus and ensures accurate assessment of uterine tone

J. Facilitates bonding

PART 2

Match the terms in Part A with a definition or related statement from Part B. Place the letter corresponding to the answer in the space provided.

PART A

1. _____ Mother's temperature is 102°F.

2. _____ Thrombophlebitis

3. _____ Urinary retention

4. _____ Mastitis

5. _____ Observing mother-child interaction

6. _____ Hemorrhage

PART B

A. Inflammation of the lining of the blood vessel

B. At each encounter

C. Provide supplementary milk for infant

D. Major danger during the immediate postoperative period

E. Urine residual greater than 100 cc after catherization

F. Infection of the breast

■ Section Two: Short Answer and Completion Exercises

PART 1

State the terms for the following definitions. Indicate your answer in the space provided.

1. _____ A time of reflection for a postpartal woman in which she is passive and wants to be ministered to

2. _____ Pink or brownish vaginal drainage noted around the fourth postpartal day

3. _____ The formation of breast milk

4. _____ The incision of the perineum made during the second stage of labor

5. _____ Exercises consisting of contracting and relaxing the muscles of the perineum

PART 2

Complete the following short answer exercises.

1. Briefly compare and contrast the taking-in, taking-hold, and letting-go postpartal phases.

2. Identify two types of rooming-in and two advantages of rooming-in.

3. List the five characteristics used to determine if lochia flow is normal.

4. Briefly describe the characteristics of "postpartal blues."

5. Explain the use of sitz bath and ice packs in the care of the postpartal woman who had an episiotomy.

PART 3

Describe the physiologic changes that occur in the indicated structures during the postpartal period.

Uterus

Cervix

Vagina

Perineum

■ Section Three: Critical Thinking for Application of Essential Concepts

PART 1

Circle the letter corresponding to the appropriate answer.

1. Mrs. Peters states that her newborn daughter Millie is so thin and has so little hair. The nurse could best help Mrs. Peters by
   A. recognizing that Mrs. Peters is feeling jealous and emphasizing that she doesn't have to find fault with the child to make herself feel attractive.
   B. acknowledging Mrs. Peters' statements, explaining that the child will grow a lot during the first months, and then pointing out many of the baby's good features and behaviors.
   C. asking Mrs. Peters if she was thin as a child and discussing the many dangers of being an underweight, malnourished newborn.
   D. discussing postpartal blues with Mrs. Peters and the fact that negative observations and thoughts are common during this time.

2. The nurse, in planning to help a woman adjust to her new baby, must consider which of the following?
   A. The mother will require little assistance since parental love is instinctive.
   B. The more difficult the labor process, the stronger the mother's bond with her child.
   C. It may be natural for the mother to be hesitant initially when touching the child.
   D. Holding the child immediately after birth is overwhelming to a new mother and should be avoided.

3. Mrs. Peters has a 4-year-old son at home and is concerned about his reaction to the new baby. The nurse might do which of the following to best assist this postpartal family?
   A. Instruct Mrs. Peters to write her son a letter and include a picture of the new baby.
   B. Encourage Mrs. Peters to have another family member spend a lot of time with her son.
   C. Arrange for the son to visit with Mrs. Peters and the baby as soon as possible.
   D. Discuss the dangers of sibling rivalry with Mrs. Peters and encourage strict discipline.

4. When examining a postpartal woman, the nurse should immediately report
   A. a fundus that is palpated 2 cm below the umbilicus on the second postpartal day.
   B. a fundus that cannot be located by palpation on the ninth postpartal day.
   C. a soft, spongy uterine fundus noted during the first hour postpartum.
   D. red, bloody vaginal discharge on the perineal pad on the first day postpartum.

5. During the postpartal period the new mother may experience an alteration in urinary elimination related to loss of bladder sensation. Which of the following data would indicate this problem?

 A. A resonant sound noted on percussion of the lower abdominal area

 B. A firm fundus located 1 cm below the umbilicus on the first postpartal day

 C. Complaints of pain at the episiotomy site, particularly after ambulation

 D. Urinary output greater than 1,500 mL during a 24-hour period

6. The nurse could encourage which of the following measures to decrease the sense of abandonment experienced by the woman and her mate during the postpartal period?

 A. The couple should plan extensive time with the new baby to increase their sense of bonding and decrease jealousy.

 B. The father should be encouraged to share in the care and feeding of the child to increase feelings of involvement.

 C. Discussions of parenting should be avoided during the immediate postpartal period to minimize anticipatory resentment.

 D. The mother should be warned that being jealous of the attention her child is receiving is a sign of postpartal psychosis.

7. Which of the following statements related to the patient's nutritional status is a common finding or recommended measure during the postpartal period?

 A. Breastfeeding mothers should limit caloric intake to prevent fat-cell buildup in newborns, which could lead to obesity.

 B. Fluid intake is limited for 48 hours due to the high fluid volume retained in the body after delivery.

 C. High intake of meats, fish, chicken, and dairy products should be encouraged to facilitate good tissue repair.

 D. The mother will have little desire for food or fluids for 24 hours due to the gluconeogenesis that occurs postpartum.

8. Which of the following is an appropriate nursing diagnosis for a postpartal mother with an episiotomy during the first 5 days postpartum?

 A. Anxiety related to vaginal scar formation and decreased body image

 B. Alteration in nutrition: more than body requirements related to increased appetite

 C. High risk for infection related to lochia and decreased perineal skin integrity

 D. Self-care deficit related to poor opportunity for independence

9. The postpartal mother asks the nurse when her body will return to "normal." The nurse should implement a teaching plan about postpartal bodily changes that includes which of the following information?

 A. A fast heart rate and thready pulse will occasionally be noted and should be expected.

 B. Menstrual flow will return within 6 to 10 weeks after delivery unless the mother is breastfeeding.

 C. Varicosities and vascular blemishes will disappear by the sixth postpartal week.

 D. The weight gained during pregnancy is usually retained regardless of dietary and exercise efforts.

10. Which of the following would be cause for concern if found during a postpartal assessment?

    A. Diaphoresis during the period immediately after delivery

    B. Hair loss over the postpartal period

    C. Pale coloring of the inner conjunctiva

    D. Reports of slight breast tenderness

11. The appropriate method for assessment of the fundus would be to

    A. massage the uterus between the thumb and middle finger until firm, then use a ruler to measure location.

    B. palpate the fundus while the woman has a full bladder to facilitate detection of the uterus.

    C. place both hands below the symphysis pubis and push upward until the lower end of the fundus is located.

    D. support the lower segment of the uterus while palpating the fundus to prevent inversion.

12. Placing the infant at the breast to breastfeed has what effect on uterine tone?

    A. Breastfeeding stimulates lactation, which increases the formation of clots in the uterus.

    B. Stimulation of the breast causes oxytocin release and decreased tone in the uterine wall.

    C. The pressure of the infant breastfeeding can cause uterine rupture.

    D. Uterine contraction is stimulated by the infant sucking on the breast.

13. Which of the following is the most appropriate outcome criterion for the postpartal mother and family?

    A. Client demonstrates the procedure for self-examination of the breast, the fundus, and perineal area and states her intent to perform these exams.

    B. Client's temperature is 100.4° to 101°F; no redness or discharge of any kind is noted during the first 48 hours after delivery.

    C. Client does not request pain medication for episiotomy pain and tolerates breast discomfort with minimal comment.

    D. Client prepares a menu including low-calorie foods and minimal intake of meats and bread or starchy food products.

14. The nurse is caring for 14-year-old Lisa, who has decided to give her baby up for adoption. Which of the following should the nurse keep in mind?

    A. Lisa would probably keep her baby if she were given encouragement.

    B. After the delivery Lisa may express a desire to keep her baby, or she may want to continue with the adoption.

    C. During the taking-in phase of the puerperium, the nurse should encourage Lisa to reconsider her decision to abandon her baby.

    D. Lisa should not hold, see, or touch her baby after the delivery to decrease her feelings of loss after giving the child away.

15. Data supporting a diagnosis of "high risk for fluid volume deficit related to subinvolution" would include

    A. blood pressure of 120/62 noted on the third day after delivery.

    B. firm uterine fundus located at standard measurement level.

C. lochia saturating one perineal pad per hour 12 hours postpartum.

D. pulse slow and bounding during the first postpartal day.

16. Which of the following nursing interventions would be appropriate when caring for an episiotomy client who has the nursing diagnosis "Pain related to perineal sutures"?

A. Apply ice packs to the perineal incision site to decrease edema.

B. Discourage client from contracting and relaxing perineal muscles.

C. Instruct client to use petroleum jelly or mineral oil on the episiotomy as desired.

D. Limit pain medication to prevent dependence on narcotic analgesics.

17. An appropriate goal for a postpartal client who complains of being exhausted and unable to sleep would be that the client

A. abstain from performing self-care and rest instead.

B. state she feels rested during the postpartal period.

C. sleep during the night in order to stay awake all day.

D. sleep 8 hours every night after discharge from the hospital.

18. A client with the diagnosis of "Self-esteem disturbance related to lack of knowledge regarding psychological changes during the postpartal period" might have which of the following defining characteristics?

A. She denies that she has feelings of abandonment or fatigue.

B. She performs grooming and infant care activities.

C. She states that she will not be jealous of her child any longer.

D. She verbalizes that she has conflicting feelings.

PART 2: CASE STUDY

Rena Despande, age 30, has just given birth to her third daughter. Her husband, age 39, states he wanted a boy but is glad both his wife and the baby are healthy. The baby weighed 10 pounds and Rena had to have an episiotomy.

1. What effect might Rena's husband's hopes for a male child have on the couple's postpartal adjustments? What nursing actions might be implemented?

2. Rena shows reluctance to touch her perineal area and resists discussing perineal care. What factors (including culture) might contribute to Rena's discomfort with performing and discussing perineal care?

■ Section Four: Inquiry and Exploration

PART 1: CRITICAL INQUIRY EXERCISES

1. Write a teaching plan that could be used to prepare new parents for the emotional and physiologic changes occurring after childbirth.

2. What suggestions would you make to a woman who states she has "no time" to perform muscle-strengthening exercises because of childcare and home care responsibilities but says she really wants to get back in shape?

PART 2: CRITICAL EXPLORATION EXERCISES

1. During a pediatric clinical experience, perform postpartal assessments on two women and compare findings related to the physiologic and psychological status of each.

2. Interview a woman and her spouse (if possible) during the immediate postpartal period. Attempt to identify signs that the following are being experienced: abandonment, disappointment, or postpartal blues.

Nursing Care of the Newborn and Family

CHAPTER OVERVIEW

Chapter 23 presents exercises to refine knowledge of newborn assessment and care. It is important that the nurse be able to evaluate findings obtained on assessment and intervene appropriately when these findings suggest underlying pathology. This chapter assists the student in recognizing "normal" findings and differentiating them from abnormal findings. Anticipatory guidance with regard to feeding, daily routines, and the characteristics of stools is addressed.

LEARNING OBJECTIVES

After mastering the contents of this chapter, you should be able to:

1. Describe the characteristics of the term newborn.

2. Assess a newborn for normal growth and development.

3. Use the nursing process to identify and address nursing diagnoses related to the newborn and/or family of the newborn.

4. Identify National Health Goals related to newborns that nurses can be instrumental in helping the nation achieve.

5. Identify areas related to newborn assessment and care that could benefit from additional nursing research.

6. Use critical thinking to analyze ways that the care of the term newborn can be more family centered.

7. Synthesize knowledge of newborn growth and development and immediate care needs with the nursing process to achieve quality maternal and child health nursing care.

KEY TERMS

acrocyanosis	hemangioma	neonate
caput succedaneum	jaundice	nevus flammeus
cavernous hemangioma	kangaroo care	physiologic jaundice
central cyanosis	kernicterus	pseudomenstruation
cephalhematoma	lanugo	radiation
conduction	meconium	strawberry hemangioma
convection	milia	subconjunctival hemorrhage
Crede treatment	mongolian spot	thrush
erythema toxicum	natal teeth	transitional stool
evaporation	neonatal period	vernix caseosa

■ Section One:
Identification of Key Terms and Concepts

PART 1

Match the terms in Part A with a definition or related statement from Part B. Place the letter corresponding to the answer in the space provided. (Use each letter only once; some letters may not be used.)

PART A

1. _____ Subconjunctival hemorrhage
2. _____ Physiologic jaundice
3. _____ Crede treatment
4. _____ Extrusion reflex
5. _____ Nevus flammeus
6. _____ Cremasteric reflex
7. _____ Strawberry hemangioma
8. _____ Brown fat
9. _____ Neonatal period
10. _____ Natal teeth

PART B

A. A special tissue found in mature newborns to conserve or produce body heat
B. Prophylaxis against gonorrheal conjunctivitis for the newborn
C. Pressure during birth causing a red spot on the sclera
D. Movement upward of the testes when the inner aspect of the thigh is stroked
E. Narrow distance between the eyes
F. Infant attempts to refuse solid foods
G. Yellowing of the skin as a result of the breakdown of fetal red blood cells
H. Port-wine stain-hemangioma lesion level with skin
I. Vascular tumor of the skin, elevated areas formed by immature capillaries and epithelial cells
J. One or two dental eruptions present at birth
K. Time from birth through the first 28 days

PART 2

Indicate if the following statements are true or false by placing a "T" or "F" in the space provided.

1. _____ Infants who do not void within 24 hours after birth could possibly have urethral stenosis.

2. _____ Murmurs heard when examining the neonate usually indicate cardiac anomalies and must be corrected surgically.

3. _____ An accelerated count of leukocytes in the newborn's serology test suggests a response to an infection.

4. _____ A circumcision prevents phimosis and reduces the incidence of urinary tract infections.

■ Section Two: Short Answer and Completion Exercises

PART 1

Complete the following fill-in-the-blank exercises.

1. The time of birth through the first 28 days of life is termed the _____

   _____.

2. The infant is vulnerable to heat instability and loses heat readily through four

   separate mechanisms: _____ , _____ , _____ and

   _____.

3. The average heart rate for the neonate is _____.

4. The average respiratory rate for the neonate is _____.

PART 2

Complete the following short answer exercises.

1. List the six criteria described by Berry Brazelton that are used as the basis to evaluate the newborn's behavioral capacity.

   _____ _____

   _____ _____

   _____ _____

2. Describe and contrast the stools of a bottle- and breast-fed infant.

3. Why would the nurse be concerned after learning that a neonate has not passed a stool at 24 hours after birth?

4. Identify the behaviors exhibited by the newborn in the following periods.

   First period of reactivity:

   Second period of reactivity:

5. Explain the principles of safety when placing a child in a car seat or car seat belt.

6. Discuss the potential adverse effects of elective surgery to the male infant's penile gland.

7. State the interventions of the nursing process to prevent postsurgical complications.

8. Explain why parents, visitors, and hospital personnel with cold sores should not care for the newborn infant.

■ Section Three:
Critical Thinking for Application of Essential Concepts

PART 1

Circle the letter corresponding to the appropriate answer.

Questions 1-5 relate to the following situation: Mrs. Lee delivered (breech) a baby boy today. You are assigned as the nurse to take care of him. Baby boy Lee was evaluated to be at 39 weeks gestation and weighed 3500 grams.

1. On baby Lee's second hospital day, the nurse performs her morning assessment. When assessing the chest comparatively to the head, she would expect
   A. the chest circumference to be about 2 cm less than the head circumference.
   B. the head and chest circumference to be equal.
   C. the head circumference to be about 2 cm less than the chest circumference.
   D. the head circumference to be about 3 cm more than the chest circumference.

2. The nurse notes that the infant's temperature is slightly subnormal an hour after birth. What would be an appropriate measure?

   A. Take the infant to the mother for bonding and transfer of body heat when possiMCAe.

   B. Place a second stockinette on the infant's head.

   C. Administer a warm bath with temperature slightly higher than usual.

   D. Place the infant under a radiant warmer or heated isolette.

3. Which of the following findings on the nurse assessment would warrant a call to the physician?

   A. Breast tissue slightly engorged

   B. Heart rate of 170 beats per minute

   C. A crepitant-like feeling when assessing the clavicals

   D. Frog-like positioning of the lower extremities

4. When listening to heart and lung sounds the nurse found all the following on auscultation. Which would suggest a pathological disturbance?

   A. Splitting of S1 increased on inspiration

   B. Bronchi sounds over the chest wall

   C. Grunting sounds when lying on abdomen

   D. Radiating sounds of mucus from the throat or the chest wall

5. The nurse attempts to elicit the Moro reflex by

   A. brushing or stroking the cheek near the corner of the mouth.

   B. loudly tapping the bassinet.

   C. audible grunting sounds.

   D. stroking the side of the feet in an attempt to have the toes spread in a "fan" fashion.

PART 2: CASE STUDY

Mrs. Calland delivered (vaginally) a baby boy today. Baby boy Calland was evaluated to be 38 weeks gestation and weigh 3200 grams. Mrs. Calland plans to breastfeed her baby. You are assigned as the nurse to take care of her and her baby.

1. Shortly after delivery a number of reflexes were tested on the infant. Make a list of reflexes that were tested and explain which maneuvers were used to complete the tests.

2. Within 12 hours after birth the infant passed a sticky black stool. Explain why this should not alarm you.

3. On the day of discharge, baby boy Calland appears to have yellow skin and sclera. What lab test might be ordered at this time? What would be indicated if the results are higher than normal values?

4. What effect does breastfeeding have on this condition?

■ Section Four: Inquiry and Exploration

PART 1: CRITICAL INQUIRY EXERCISES

1. Formulate a nursing care plan that will focus on nursing care for a male infant who has difficulty maintaining an appropriate body temperature.

2. Develop a neonatal admission assessment form that might be used in a newborn nursery.

PART 2: CRITICAL EXPLORATION EXERCISES

1. Identify a mother who has just given birth to her first child. Formulate a teaching plan that will focus on immediate care needs for the newborn in the home environment. Discuss this information with the mother and include the father of the child, if he is available.

2. Locate the resources in your community that help families obtain car seats when they cannot afford to buy one.

3. Identify a newborn infant who is more than 24 hours old. Perform the Brazelton Neonatal Behavioral Assessment and present your findings to the class.

Nutritional Needs of the Newborn

CHAPTER OVERVIEW

Chapter 24 reviews the nutritional needs of the newborn. The nutrients in breast milk and commercially prepared formulas are evaluated and contrasted. The physiology of good nutrition is important for the growth and development of the newborn infant. After reading this chapter the student should know how to assess and evaluate the mother's ability to feed the infant and the infant's response to nutritional intake. The chapter also enables the student to provide nursing care for the mother and infant using a nursing care plan as a teaching tool.

LEARNING OBJECTIVES

After mastering the contents of this chapter, you should be able to:

1. Describe nutritional requirements of the term newborn.

2. Assess the nutritional intake of a newborn to determine adequate nutritional status.

3. Formulate nursing diagnoses related to newborn nutrition.

4. Identify appropriate outcomes for the newborn and mother related to nutrition.

5. Plan a method of infant feeding with a mother that will be satisfying for both her and the infant.

6. Implement or help parents implement feeding procedures with newborn infants.

7. Evaluate outcomes for achievement and effectiveness of care.

8. Identify National Health Goals related to newborn nutrition that nurses can be instrumental in helping the nation achieve.

9. Identify areas related to nutrition and newborns that could benefit from additional nursing research or application of evidence-based practice.

10. Use critical thinking to assist mothers with nutritional problem solving and making newborn nutrition more family-centered.

11. Integrate the knowledge of normal newborn nutrition with the nursing process to achieve quality maternal and child health nursing care.

KEY TERMS

areola
bifidus factor
colostrum
engorgement
foremilk
hind milk

interferon
lactiferous sinuses
lactoferrin
let-down reflex
lysozyme
prolactin

■ Section One:
Identification of Key Terms and Concepts

PART 1

Match the terms in Part A with a definition or related statement from Part B. Place the letter corresponding to the answer in the space provided.

PART A

1. _____ Adrenocorticosteroid hormone

2. _____ Lactose

3. _____ Histidine

4. _____ Lactiferous sinuses

6. _____ Oxytocin hormone

7. _____ IgA

8. _____ Soap

9. _____ Casein

10. _____ Colostrum

11. _____ Nipple rolling

12. _____ Lysozyme

13. _____ Hind milk

14. _____ Carbohydrates

15. _____ Fluoride

PART B

A. Finds large molecules of foreign proteins including viruses and bacteria; prohibits absorption through the gastrointestinal tract

B. Probably plays a role in assisting mammary glands to secrete milk

C. Hormone of the posterior pituitary gland that aids in uterine contractions

D. Procedure used in preparation for breast-feeding to stimulate nipple to protrude and remove adhesions

E. An amino acid essential for infant growth found in human breast milk and cow's milk

F. Contraindicated when breast-feeding; tends to cause the nipples to dry and crack

G. Thin, watery, yellow fluid consisting of protein, sugar, fat, water, minerals, vitamins, and maternal antibodies

H. Reservoirs for breast milk located behind nipple

I. The protein in cow's milk

J. Allows protein to be used for building of new cells rather than for calories

K. Necessary mineral for building sound teeth and resistance to tooth decay

L. An enzyme that aids in destroying bacteria by dissolving their cell membranes

M. "New milk" formed after the let-down reflex

N. Sugar nutrients found in breast milk that provide ready glucose for rapid brain growth

O. A fatty acid not found in skim milk but is necessary for growth and skin integrity in infants

PART 2

Indicate if the following statements are true or false by placing a "T" or "F" in the space provided.

1. _____ Infants who are fed by propping the bottles are in potential danger of aspirating fluids.

2. _____ Infants put to bed with a bottle of milk risk developing "baby bottle syndrome."

3. _____ If a woman is experiencing sore nipples from breastfeeding, she should use a hand pump to express the milk manually until the nipples have had a chance to heal.

4. _____ Colostrum is the primary constituent of breast milk during the first 3 months of feeding.

5. _____ Oxytocin is released by breastfeeding and stimulates contractions.

6. _____ The more often breasts are emptied, the more efficiently they will fill and continue to maintain a good supply of milk.

7. _____ Placing the breastfed infant over one shoulder and gently stroking his or her back is the best position for burping him or her.

8. _____ Sore nipples are a contraindication for breastfeeding.

▪ Section Two: Short Answer and Completion Exercises

Complete the following exercises relating to the physiology of breast milk production.

1. _____ milk is produced by the alveolar cells of the _____ gland in the presence of the hormone prolactin.

2. _____ _____ _____ _____ allows progesterone levels to drop and stimulates the production of the _____ hormone.

3. The infant promotes continuous milk production by _____.

4. Prolactin-releasing factor stimulates the _____ _____ ,
   which responds with active production of _____.

5. For the woman who might be experiencing preterm labor, nipple rolling is
   contraindicated because _____

   _____ .

■ Section Three:
Critical Thinking for Application of Essential Concepts

PART 1

Circle the letter corresponding to the appropriate answer.

Jane Albright is breastfeeding her baby girl, whom she delivered at 6 this morning,
weighing 6 lb 7.5 oz. The labor and delivery for mother and infant were
uneventful.

1. During the first feeding, Mrs. Albright asked how long her baby should suck
   on each breast per feeding. The nurse's best response would be which of the
   following?
   A. The infant should start nursing about 15 minutes on each breast.
   B. Five minutes on each breast for each feeding will be sufficient for today.
   C. Nurse only on one breast today for 5 minutes per feeding and start
      alternating breasts with the first feeding tomorrow.
   D. Ten minutes at each breast will be sufficient and will also keep the infant
      from becoming fatigued.

2. When counseling Mrs. Albright on breastfeeding, the nurse would know that
   the most fundamental ingredient for success is
   A. to teach Mrs. Albright how to relax.
   B. placing the infant correctly on the breast.
   C. teaching Mrs. Albright how to hold the infant in the various feeding
      positions.
   D. waiting until the infant actively demands a feeding.

3. On the second postpartum day, the nurse observes Mrs. Albright washing her
   breast and hands with soap just before she is to receive her infant for the next
   feeding. The nurse's action, if any, would be governed by which of the follow-
   ing statements?
   A. Good hygiene is necessary when breastfeeding to avoid the spread of
      pathogens from the mother's skin to the newborn.
   B. Mrs. Albright should not clean her breast and hands in preparation for
      feeding until the infant has arrived in the room.
   C. Cleansing the breast with soap may lead to nipple soreness and dryness.
   D. Stimulating the breast with washing produces increased activity of milk
      production that may be wastefully expressed before the infant is to be fed.

4. On the third postpartum day, Mrs. Albright tells the nurse that she sometimes has difficulty getting the infant to suck. She describes the infant opening her mouth when the breast touches her face but turning her head in the opposite direction. The nurse would explain that this behavior is related to

   A. the infant's immaturity and unfamiliarity with the technique of feeding.

   B. the extrusion reflex, which is normal for newborns and demonstrates the need for much assistance to ensure adequate nutrition.

   C. the rooting reflex, which suggests improper technique when placing the infant on the breast.

   D. turning neck reflex, which suggests that breastfed infants are most sensitive to tactile stimulation.

5. Mrs. Albright reports that her daughter often falls asleep at feedings before she has taken in enough nutrients. Which of the following statements would be a helpful suggestion?

   A. Wash the infant's face with cool water.

   B. Give the infant a bath before alternating breasts to complete the feeding.

   C. Rub the fontanel of the infant's head gently.

   D. Tickle the bottom of the infant's feet.

6. Which of the following preparations of commercial formulas is the least expensive?

   A. Powder to be combined with water

   B. Condensed liquid to be diluted with equal parts of water

   C. "Ready to pour" type

   D. Individually prepackaged

7. Choose the correct statement to be used to calculate a nutrient needed for the newborn infant.

   A. Fluid needs are approximately 100 cc/kg body weight/day.

   B. Fat needs are approximately 20 g/kg body weight/day.

   C. Protein needs are 2.2 g/kg body weight/day.

   D. Caloric needs are 100 kcal/kg body weight/day.

8. Which of the following is an acceptable guideline for use and storage of canned formula?

   A. The nutrients in canned formula may be enhanced with whole milk.

   B. Spring water in most instances is found to be clean and more suitable in preparing infant formula.

   C. Refrigerating unused portions of the infant's formula after feedings is a good practice.

   D. Formula in an open can should be used or discarded in 24 hours.

PART 2: CASE STUDY

Ms. Jackson delivered an 8-lb, 6-oz baby girl about 1 hour before your arrival to the clinical site this morning. Your instructor has assigned you to Ms. Jackson for the next 2 days of your clinical rotation. Her prenatal record indicates that she was considering breastfeeding but had not decided at the time of birth. You will need to be prepared to answer her questions about breastfeeding.

1. Compare the advantages and disadvantages of breast-feeding for the infant and mother.

2. What are some appropriate measures to relieve breast engorgement?

3. State how the infant should be properly placed on the breast for feeding.

4. What are some common reasons why breastfed infants do not suck well?

■ Section Four: Inquiry and Exploration

PART 1: CRITICAL INQUIRY EXERCISES

1. Mrs. Jones' water supply is furnished by her private well. She will be preparing formula for her newborn infant. Outline the steps of sterilization to teach her how to prepare the formula and supplement.

2. Design a teaching tool for parents about the techniques and safeguards of feeding for breast- and bottle-fed babies.

PART 2: CRITICAL EXPLORATION EXERCISES

1. Survey your community for agencies that promote infant nutrition and parental education. After compiling the list, inform your clients of these agencies before their discharge.

2. Review the nursing care plans in your clinical areas for a mother and infant scheduled for discharge planning at your hospital. Note the information pertinent to infant nutrition. Exercise your teaching skills by providing this information to a parent the day before discharge. On the day of discharge, assess the effectiveness of your teaching by interviewing your client. Create your own evaluation tool.

CHAPTER 25

Nursing Care of the Woman and Family Experiencing a Postpartal Complication

CHAPTER OVERVIEW

A woman experiencing a postpartal complication is subject to difficulty in bonding with her child. If the illness responds poorly to treatment, her potential to give birth to another child may be threatened. Many postpartal complications can be prevented with the support of a health team's assessment skills and the ability of each professional caring for the postpartal patient to evaluate findings and intervene appropriately.

LEARNING OBJECTIVES

After mastering the contents of this chapter, you should be able to:

1. Describe common deviations from the normal that can occur during the puerperium.

2. Assess the woman and her family for deviations from the normal during the puerperium.

3. Identify and address nursing diagnoses related to deviations from the normal during the puerperium.

4. Identify National Health Goals related to postpartal complications that nurses can be instrumental in helping the nation achieve.

5. Identify areas related to complications during the puerperium that could benefit from additional nursing research.

6. Use critical thinking to analyze ways that the care of the woman experiencing a postpartal complication can be more family-centered.

7. Synthesize knowledge of postpartal complications with the nursing process to achieve quality maternal and child health nursing care.

KEY TERMS

endometritis
mastitis
peritonitis
postpartal depression
postpartal psychosis
Sheehan's syndrome
thrombophlebitis

■ Section One:
Identification of Key Terms and Concepts

PART 1

Match the terms in Part A with a definition or related statement from Part B. Place the letter corresponding to the answer in the space provided.

PART A

1. _____ Thrombophlebitis

2. _____ Endometritis

3. _____ Perineal hematomas

4. _____ Postpartal depression

5. _____ Peritonitis

6. _____ Urinary retention

7. _____ Mastitis

PART B

A. A collection of blood in the subcutaneous layer of the perineum
B. Infection of the breast
C. Induced by edema of the bladder from pressures during childbirth
D. Emotional feeling of sadness related to hormonal changes
E. Inflammation of the lining of a blood vessel with the formation of blood clots
F. Infection of the peritoneal cavity
G. Infection of the lining of the uterus

PART 2

Indicate if the following statements are true or false by placing a "T" or "F" in the space provided.

1. _____ The majority of the complications occurring during the puerperium are preventable.

2. _____ Women who experience blood loss greater than 500 cc in 24 hours are traditionally considered to be hemorrhaging and may require blood replacement.

3. _____ An elevated level of human chorionic gonadotropin (hCG) is present if the postpartal woman has retained placental fragments after the birth of the placenta.

4. _____ Most postpartal infections are caused by staphylococcal organisms.

■ Section Two: Short Answer and Completion Exercises

PART 1

Complete the following short answer exercises.

1. List the four reasons that are most often found to be the precipitating causes of postpartal hemorrhage.

   _____   _____

   _____   _____

2. Define disseminated intravascular coagulation (DIC).

3. What are the common causes of DIC during the postpartal period?

4. Identify the cardinal signs of postpartal-induced hypertension.

PART 2

Complete the following short answer exercises.

1. What is the rationale that supports teaching women to wipe the perineal area from front to back when cleansing or removing feces?

2. What is considered to be an accurate account of measuring blood loss from lochia?

3. What observational technique can be practiced in assessing lochia to detect a cervical tear that occurred during the birthing process?

4. Endometritis is a preventable postpartal complication that may lead to a more serious illness. What are the important components of the nurse's assessment to determine the early signs of endometritis?

5. Explain why it is important to inspect the placenta after an uncomplicated delivery.

■ Section Three:
Critical Thinking for Application of Essential Concepts

PART 1

Circle the letter corresponding to the appropriate answer.

1. Which of the following symptoms suggests a postpartal complication?
   A. Lochia rubra 12 hours after birth
   B. Temperature of 100.4°F or less
   C. Blood loss of more than 12 oz/24 hrs
   D. 20 to 24 sanitary pads saturated/24 hrs

2. Mrs. Jones is experiencing signs of shock about 3 hours after delivery. Which of the symptoms below will the nurse expect to find on assessing Mrs. Jones?
   A. Increase in diastolic blood pressure > 10 mm Hg
   B. Decrease in pulse rate
   C. Rapid respirations
   D. Flushed face

3. The physician determines Mrs. Jones is hemorrhaging from uterine atony. The nurse may expect to administer
   A. Apresoline.
   B. Zaroxolyn.
   C. Methergine.
   D. Proventil.

4. What is the most important action to be taken by the nurse in reference to a postpartal client who has significant blood loss?
   A. Assess the chart record for type and cross-matching results.
   B. Assess the chart for any record of ABO incompatibility.
   C. Immediately obtain a blood specimen for a hematocrit and hemoglobin.
   D. Place the client in a semi-Fowler's position with the extremities elevated.

5. Which of the following is viewed as a precursor of a postpartal infection?

   A. Thyroid toxicosis

   B. Excessive blood loss

   C. Pregnancy-induced hypertension

   D. Negative Rh factor

6. What is an appropriate measure in caring for the client who has experienced a fourth-degree laceration of the perineum?

   A. Encourage her to douche at least once a week to reduce organisms that may come in contact with the perineal area.

   B. Administer analgesic rectal suppositories to promote comfort.

   C. Encourage fluid intake and foods high in fiber.

   D. Administer an enema when necessary to prevent constipation.

■ PART 2: Case Study

Mrs. Lawson, age 36, gravida 3 para 3, is suffering from a puerperal infection during the postpartum period. You are assigned to work with Mrs. Lawson on the sixth day of her hospital stay.

1. What would be considered a probable cause of Mrs. Lawson's condition?

2. Are there any measures that could have been considered to avoid this illness? As you review Mrs. Lawson's records you find that her assessment, several days ago, revealed data that may have suggested the beginning of her present illness.

3. What are some indicators that patients presenting with Mrs. Lawson's illness often exhibit?

4. Discuss the therapeutic measures that will be used to assist this patient.

■ Section Four: Inquiry and Exploration

PART 1: CRITICAL INQUIRY EXERCISES

1. Prepare a discharge teaching packet for a client with thrombophlebitis.

2. Consider the risk of exposure to an infection during delivery. Develop a set of guidelines that can serve as protective measures against the development of endometritis.

PART 2: CRITICAL EXPLORATION EXERCISES

Review the policy of the agency where you are doing your maternal health clinical rotation. Identify the ward's policy on the nurse's authority to order blood from the blood bank for a client who is experiencing a postpartal hemorrhage.

CHAPTER 26

Nursing Care of the High-Risk Newborn and Family

CHAPTER OVERVIEW

The high-risk neonate may have difficulty establishing respirations at birth. This newborn will need care from a skilled professional health team. The neonate's problem may be related to gestational age, physiologic complications, pregnancy complications, or unhealthy maternal lifestyle. After completion of this chapter the student will be able to care for the high-risk newborn who needs resuscitation and maintenance of respiration.

LEARNING OBJECTIVES

After mastering the contents of this chapter, you should be able to:

1. Define essential terms related to the gestational ages of infants.

2. Assess a high-risk newborn in the early neonatal period to determine if the infant has completed a safe transition to extrauterine life.

3. Formulate a nursing care plan for an infant classified as high risk.

4. Describe the characteristics of infants born with low birthweights and who are small or large for gestational age.

5. Use critical thinking to analyze the special crisis imposed on families when alterations of newborn development, length of pregnancy, or neonatal illness occur.

6. Synthesize knowledge of the needs of the high-risk infant with the nursing process to achieve quality maternal and child health nursing care.

KEY TERMS

apnea
apparent life-threatening event
appropriate for gestational age
brown fat
caudal regression syndrome
cephalopelvic disproportion
developmental care
dysmature
extracorporeal membrane
  oxygenation (ECMO)
extremely-very-low-birthweight
  infant
gestational age

hemorrhagic disease of
  the newborn
hydrops fetalis
hyperbilirubinemia
hyperglycemia
hypocalcemia
hypoglycemia
intrauterine growth retardation
kernicterus
large-for-gestational-age infant
low-birthweight infant
macrosomia
ophthalmia neonatorum

periodic respirations
periventricular leukomalacia
postterm infant
postterm syndrome
preterm infant
primary apnea
retinopathy of prematurity
secondary apnea
shoulder dystocia
small-for-gestational-age infant
term infant
transient tachypnea
very-low-birthweight infant

▪ Section One:
Identification of Key Terms and Concepts

PART 1

Match the period of fetal-newborn life in Part A with the most common type of infections contracted during that period in Part B. Place the letter corresponding to the answer in the space provided.

PART A

1. _____ Prenatal

2. _____ Perinatal

3. _____ Postnatal

PART B

A. Contracted through contact with infected hospital worker

B. Cytomegalovirus or toxoplasmosis viral infection

C. Group B streptococcal septicemia, thrush, or herpes

PART 2

Match the age or weight classification in Part A with the description of the infant in Part B.

PART A

1. _____ Term

2. _____ Low birthweight

3. _____ Postterm

4. _____ Small for gestational age

5. _____ Large for gestational age

PART B

A. Infant whose weight falls below the tenth percentile of weight for gestational age

B. Infant whose weight falls above the ninetieth percentile of weight for age

C. Infant born between 30 and 36 weeks' gestation (birthweight less than 2,500 g)

D. Infant born after the onset of week 43 of pregnancy

E. Infant born after week 38 or before week 43 of pregnancy

PART 3

Indicate if the following statements are true or false by placing a "T" or "F" in the space provided.

1. _____ A newborn's attempt to raise his or her body temperature increases his or her need for oxygen.

2. _____ A newborn's attempt to raise his or her body temperature increases his or her metabolic rate.

3. _____ ypercalcemia is a common nutritional problem of the small-for-gestational-age infant.

4. _____ Infants of drug-dependent mothers become symptomatic approximately 48 hours after birth.

■ Section Two: Short Answer and Completion Exercises

PART 1

Complete the following short answer exercises.

1. Describe the respiratory pattern of primary apnea.

2. Discuss two causes of intrauterine growth retardation and state one example of each.

3. Explain the concept of extracorporeal membrane oxygenation (ECMO).

4. What is the rationale for administering vitamin E to a premature infant with anemia?

5. Define kernicterus.

6. Discuss how periodic respiration differs from true apnea and periodic apnea.

7. Why is the immediate administration of oxygen under pressure (bag and mask) contraindicated for infants who are born with meconium-stained amniotic fluid?

8. Discuss the physiology of transient tachypnea.

PART 2

Complete the following short answer and fill-in-the-blank exercises.

1. What are the eight priority areas of nursing care that are most often linked to the illnesses of infants with altered gestational ages?

2. Retinopathy of prematurity (ROP) is an acquired ocular disease that leads to _____ and is caused by _____ of immature retinal blood vessels.

■ Section Three:
Critical Thinking for Application of Essential Concepts

PART 1

Circle the letter corresponding to the appropriate answer.

1. Baby girl LaTrond is born with an Apgar score of 5 and 7. The infant is experiencing respiratory difficulty. The nurse's immediate goal for this infant would be to
   A. establish adequate circulatory pattern within 2 minutes.
   B. clear the airway and establish respirations in 2 minutes.
   C. prevent respiratory distress syndrome.
   D. obtain the oxygen concentration in the circulating blood volume.

2. The nurse would know that failure to obtain this immediate goal may result in
   A. respiratory alkalosis.
   B. Duchenne-Erb syndrome.
   C. respiratory acidosis.
   D. occlusion of the foramen ovale.

3. After therapeutic interventions, baby LaTrond is able to adequately expand her lungs. The amount of pressure that would enable her to continue to reinflate the alveoli of her lungs would be
   A. 6 to 10 cm of water.
   B. 8 to 12 cm of water.
   C. 10 to 15 cm of water.
   D. 15 to 20 cm of water.

4. Which of the following clinical practices is appropriate to solicit initial respirations of the high-risk newborn?
   A. Spanking the buttocks
   B. Slapping the face
   C. Squeezing the thorax
   D. Rubbing the back

5. Baby Susan is about 21 hours old and has become respiratory compromised after an uneventful delivery and "normal" newborn assessment. The nurse's initial response would be to
   A. obtain blood gas levels and position the infant prone.
   B. increase the flow of oxygen and position the infant in Trendelenburg position.
   C. position the infant on her abdomen and lower the head of the bed.
   D. position the infant with the head of the bed elevated.

6. An infant who is exposed to continuous subnormal body temperatures has a potential to develop

    A. compensatory profuse pulmonary perfusion.

    B. pulmonary alkalosis.

    C. anaerobic glycolysis.

    D. hydrops fetalis.

7. An infant whose temperature is being maintained by a radiant heat source should have the probe or disk placed

    A. over a scapula area near the midscapula line.

    B. on the abdomen between the umbilicus and the xiphoid process.

    C. over the rib cage between the costal structures.

    D. over the diaphragm below the lungs.

8. Baby girl Lathasa was born large for gestational age. After being delivered vaginally, this infant should be carefully assessed for

    A. increased intracranial pressure.

    B. hypothermia.

    C. decreased red blood levels (anemia).

    D. hyperglycemia.

9. An infant of a diabetic mother may have which of the following behavioral and characteristic appearances?

    A. Shrill, high-pitched cry

    B. Trembles, jittery, and irritable

    C. Fat, puffy, cushingoid face

    D. Overall wasting, sunken abdomen

10. On the third hospital day in the nursery, Mr. and Mrs. Hubbard's newborn baby girl Rhonda is diagnosed with Rh incompatibility. Mrs. Hubbard is a gravida 2, para 1, abortion 1. This disease causes blood cell hemolysis that is probably directly due to

    A. the exchange of fetal and maternal blood in utero.

    B. Rh-positive fetus and Rh-positive father.

    C. Rh-negative mother, Rh-positive father.

    D. the sin of the abortion of the first child.

11. Which of the following newborn characteristics would suggest that there was nutritional deprivation during fetal growth?

    A. Widely separate sutures

    B. Excessive lanugo

    C. Excessive brown fat

    D. Disproportionately small head to large body

12. When administering intravenous fluids to a high-risk infant, the nurse should be cautious to avoid which of the following?

    A. Congestive heart failure

    B. Polycythemia

    C. Decreased intracranial hemorrhage

    D. Increased tissue perfusion

PART 2: CASE STUDY

Mr. and Mrs. Boyd came to the hospital with Mrs. Boyd in active labor. She was 31 weeks pregnant and laboratory studies revealed an acute urinary tract infection. Fetal heart tones indicated fetal distress and Mrs. Boyd was prepared for a cesarean section. The Boyds had decided that the name of a male child would be Roy. Roy was born with an Apgar score of 4 and 6, weighing 1,980 g, and is preterm and small for gestational age. Six hours after birth, Baby Roy's assessment reveals severe acrocyanosis, progressive metabolic disturbances, hematocrit of 56, and specific gravity of 1.005. The infant is in severe respiratory distress and his urinary output is 1 mL/kg/hr.

1. What types of circumstances are likely to contribute to Roy's respiratory distress (for example, related to method of delivery, maternal disease, newborn condition)?

2. What initial nursing actions would be implemented to address Roy's respiratory distress, and why?

3. Why might the physician order a plasma expander for Roy, and what nursing actions would be important when administering intravenous fluids to Roy?

4. Roy has to be intubated. Formulate a plan of care for the Boyd family identifying three nursing diagnoses to facilitate parent-infant bonding and listing the nursing order.

■ Section Four: Inquiry and Exploration

PART 1: CRITICAL INQUIRY EXERCISES

1. Write a plan identifying the methods you would use to teach the mother how to implement a stimulation program at home for the preterm infant who has been deprived of environmental stimuli.

2. Identify all supporting devices and therapeutic procedures that might be used in direct support of an infant with respiratory distress syndrome. Synthesize how the devices and the procedures function to correct the pathologic processes demonstrated by assessment data and lab values.

PART 2: CRITICAL EXPLORATION EXERCISES

1. Identify a preterm infant in the high-risk nursery. Examine the prenatal history and inpatient chart. Identify any existing factors that may have precipitated an early delivery.

2. Collaborate with two of your classmates to practice the sequential steps of external cardiac massage in the newborn using the cardiopulmonary resuscitation doll. Present your skill to the class and instructors with the assistance of your two partners.

UNIT VI

The Nursing Role in Health Promotion for the Childrearing Family

Principles of Growth and Development

CHAPTER OVERVIEW

Chapter 27 examines and summarizes the basic concepts of hereditary and environmental factors that influence a child's growth and development. The theories of development according to Freud, Erikson, Piaget, and Kohlberg are discussed. The chapter also explores the developmental tasks of parenting as the child progresses through various growth stages. The implications of growth and development for the nursing care of children from various age groups are explored, and interviewing and therapeutic communication skills needed by the nurse when caring for children in various stages of growth and development are also discussed. A case study presents a contrasting view of the developmental characteristics for each stage.

LEARNING OBJECTIVES

After mastering the contents of this chapter, you should be able to:

1. Describe principles of growth and development and developmental stages according to major theorists.

2. Assess a child to determine the stage of development the child has reached.

3. Formulate nursing diagnoses that address wellness as well as both a potential for and an actual delay in growth and development.

4. Identify expected outcomes for nursing goals for a growing child.

5. Plan nursing interventions to assist a child in achieving and maintaining normal growth and development.

6. Implement nursing actions such as providing age-appropriate play materials to support normal growth and development patterns.

7. Evaluate outcomes to be certain that nursing goals related to growth and development have been achieved.

8. Identify National Health Goals related to growth and development that nurses can be instrumental in helping the nation to achieve.

9. Identify areas of nursing care related to growth and development that could benefit from additional nursing research or application of evidence-based practice.

10. Use critical thinking to analyze factors that influence growth and development and ways to strengthen paths to achieving a new developmental stage.

11. Integrate knowledge of growth and development with nursing process to achieve quality maternal and child health nursing care.

KEY TERMS

abstract thought
accommodation
adaptability
approach
assimilation
attention span
autonomy versus shame
centering
cognitive development
concrete operational thought
conservation
conventional development
development
developmental milestone

developmental task
distractibility
egocentrism
formal operational thought
growth
identity versus role confusion
industry versus inferiority
initiative versus guilt
intuitive thought
libido
macronutrient
maturation
micronutrient
mood quality

permanence
postconventional development
preoperational thought
prereligious stage
reversibility
rhythmicity
role fantasy
schema
sensorimotor stage
temperament
theory
threshold of response
trust versus mistrust

■ Section One:
Identification of Key Terms and Concepts

PART 1

*Match the terms in Part A with a definition or related statement from Part B. Place
the letter corresponding to the answer in the space provided.*

PART A

1. _____ Genetic makeup

2. _____ Temperament

3. _____ Parent-child relationship

4. _____ Latent phase

5. _____ Socioeconomic level

6. _____ Postconventional development

PART B

A. A time in which a child's libido is diverted into concrete thinking

B. May affect parents' ability to provide adequate health care and nutrition

C. A child's inherited background

D. A stage of cognitive development displayed by adolescents as they begin to
   have abstract thoughts about standards of conduct

E. An individual child's particular manner of thinking, behaving, or reacting to
   environmental stimuli

F. Loss of this crucial environmental influence can interfere with a child's growth
   and development.

PART 2

Match the following stages of Piaget's theories on development in Part A with the appropriate description of each stage in Part B. Place the letter corresponding to the answer in the space provided (more than one letter may be used for each answer).

PART A

1. _____ Sensorimotor

2. _____ Tertiary circular reaction

3. _____ Preoperational thought

4. _____ Intuitive thought

5. _____ Concrete operational thought

6. _____ Formal operational thought

PART B

A. Thoughts of what could be rather than what currently exists

B. Inductive reasoning, from specific to general

C. Relates to the environment through his or her senses, using reflex behavior

D. Concept of accommodation, the ability to modify ideas to fit reality

E. Centering, seeing only one characteristic of a given object

F. Permanency of objects in the environment

G. Objects are separate from the individual and permanent in the environment

H. Concept of conservation, matter does not change in size when moved to a different environment

I. Egotistic thought, perceives one's own thoughts and needs as more important than those of others

J. Ability to think through actions or mentally project what the solution to a problem will be, "invention of new means"

K. Draws conclusion from obvious facts only, prelogical reasoning

PART 3

Complete the following fill-in-the-blank exercises.

1. _____ and _____ are essential physical data when making an assessment and should be accurately plotted on a growth chart.

2. _____ is a synonym for development.

3. _____ is a term used to express an increase in physical size or a quantitative change.

4. _____ denotes an increase in skill or the ability to function.

5. _____ _____ includes provision of information regarding further expectation of a child's ability to function in his/her environment.

6. _____ is a term used to describe the child's intellectual abilities.

■ Section Two: Short Answer and Completion Exercises

PART 1

Complete the chart by naming the five psychoanalytic stages of development as defined by Sigmund Freud. Assign the appropriate childhood division and age range to these stages (see example).

Stage	*Childhood Division*	*Age Range*
1. Oral stage	infant	1 month to 1 year
2.		
3.		
4.		
5.		

PART 2

Identify the psychosocial stage of development that is described by each of the following statements.

1. _____ Strives to obtain a sense of independence, taking pride in new accomplishments and wanting to do everything for himself/herself

2. _____ Expends effort to gain a sense of identity, bringing together experiences previously learned

3. _____ Concentrates on perfecting learned skills while seeking to enlarge his or her environment with school and community

4. _____ Recognizes that needs are met as they arise, with discomfort being quickly removed

5. _____ Learns how to do things, and the need for freedom and opportunity to initiate motor skills increases

PART 3

State the appropriate stage of moral development described in the sentences below.

1. _____ Imitates behavior and practices doing gestures only for gestures in return

2. _____ Internalizes standards of conduct, doing what he or she thinks is right regardless of an existing social rule

3. _____ Learns that certain actions may elicit positive or negative behaviors from parents

4. _____ Punishment-obedience orientation, governed easily by parental authority

5 _____ Behaviors are influenced more by what is "nice" than by what may be right or wrong

■ Section Three:
Critical Thinking for Application of Essential Concepts

PART 1

Circle the letter corresponding to the appropriate answer.

1. Mrs. Peters complains that her daughter Millie, age 1 month, is very fussy and will not sit in her car seat. She states that Millie never responds well to new people or toys. The nurse should explain which of the following to Mrs. Peters?

   A. When children are ill they are often fussy and respond poorly to new stimuli; these children often need to be hospitalized.

   B. Children have different approaches to life, and some children naturally demonstrate withdrawal when faced with new stimuli.

   C. The behavior she described is a sign of Millie's rhythmicity and activity level, which are inborn reactivity patterns.

   D. Infants are seldom adaptable to new stimuli; as time passes Millie will probably have a less intense reaction to stimuli.

2. Jason is 2 months old. His mother reports that he wiggles and squirms constantly in his crib and wakes up at different times every day. The nurse recognizes these behaviors as examples of which of the following reaction patterns?

   A. Adaptability and attention span

   B. Distractibility and approach

   C. Mood and reaction intensity

   D. Activity and rhythmicity

3. The nurse may discuss which of the following facts about the temperament reactivity patterns of children?

   A. Early training and instruction can correct a child's apprehensive approach to new stimuli.

   B. Even children with poor adaptability can be expected to become accustomed to a new environment by the third exposure to the area.

   C. While some children will accept a substitute toy when crying for their favorite toy, others may refuse to accept anything else.

   D. Children who spend only 1 to 2 minutes with a toy before wanting a new one are usually mentally ill and sociopathic to a small degree.

4. When discussing care for Winston, who is 15 months old, with his mother, the nurse should consider the developmental tasks of parenting for which of the following divisions of childhood?

   A. Toddler

   B. Neonate

   C. Infant

   D. Preschooler

5. The nurse might discuss which of the following with the parents of Ida, a 2-year-old, during a parenting workshop?

   A. Ida can be expected to be cooperative and easily controlled at this stage of development.

   B. Ida may prefer finger foods and clothing she can put on without assistance at this age.

   C. Expect Ida to want to be held and cuddled a great deal at this stage of her development.

   D. At this age, Ida will take the initiative in activities and will question everything.

6. The parents of an adolescent

   A. must set strict limits on activities to prevent the child from becoming independent and taking initiative.

   B. often experience difficulty in becoming independent of their child's life and in developing their own interests again.

   C. should not offer support or help to the child during this stage, so a sense of independence can be developed by the child.

   D. must take an active part in planning the child's daily activities and future experiences.

7. A key developmental task of parenting is learning to determine if their child is crying from hunger, discomfort, or some other reason. This task is most important for parents of a(n):

   A. preschooler.

   B. infant.

   C. toddler.

   D. school-age child.

8. The nurse would determine that the parents of a preschooler had achieved their developmental tasks if which of the following behaviors were noted?

    A. The mother and father alternate attending kindergarten with the child each day.

    B. The child is allowed to play without limits in the home to encourage free expression and growth.

    C. The mother or father sits with the child and sips imaginary tea from a toy teacup.

    D. The child is punished for talking too much and asking too many questions.

9. An appropriate nursing diagnosis in the care of a 4-month-old child hospitalized with a respiratory tract infection and placed on strict bed rest might be:

    A. High risk for altered development related to decreased stimulation.

    B. Altered growth status related to decreased opportunity for initiative development.

    C. High risk for increased development related to exposure to varied stimuli.

    D. Altered development related to poor opportunity for independence.

10. An appropriate patient goal when caring for a 4-year-old hospitalized child might be:

    A. The child will demonstrate initiative, within limits, evidenced by asking for paper and crayons to draw a picture.

    B. The parents will demonstrate appropriate parenting task achievement by dressing and feeding the child each day.

    C. The child will demonstrate formal operational thought by discussing the importance of being in the hospital.

    D. The parents will demonstrate the ability to interpret the child's behavioral cues.

PART 2: CASE STUDY

Consider the most recent pediatric patient for whom you have provided nursing care in the clinical environment. Note the cognitive, psychosocial, and moral stages of the child's development.

1. Write a summary of the characteristics that you were able to identify for each of these stages. Include how the patient demonstrated each stage of development.

2. Indicate whether the stage of development was appropriate for the child's chronologic age.

3. Evaluate your assessment by writing a rationale as to why you think the patient did or did not meet the developmental task for each of the stages.

■ Section Four: Inquiry and Exploration

PART 1: CRITICAL INQUIRY EXERCISES

1. Write a teaching plan that could be used to prepare the parent of a 13-month-old for the next stage of the child's development.

2. Compile a list of potentially dangerous areas in the average household environment that would be accessible to a toddler. Write to the nearest pediatric hospital's education department to obtain information that they provide to their clients and families on safety and anticipatory guidance.

PART 2: CRITICAL EXPLORATION EXERCISES

Choose a stage of childhood and interview a parent with a child in that age range. Attempt to identify the type of temperament reactivity pattern manifested by the child in each of the nine categories and evidence that the parent has, or has not, met the developmental tasks of parenting for the child's developmental stage.

CHAPTER 28

The Family With an Infant

CHAPTER OVERVIEW

This chapter discusses the growth and development patterns of the infant and family. Emphasis is placed on specific growth and development parameters and common health deviations that should be assessed during routine child health visits. Nursing interventions aimed at family support, anticipatory guidance, and alleviating common health problems are highlighted. The case study explores appropriate interventions and rationales during a well-child visit in a health facility.

LEARNING OBJECTIVES

After mastering the contents of this chapter, you should be able to:

1. Describe normal infant growth and development and associated parental concerns.

2. Assess an infant for normal growth and development milestones.

3. Formulate nursing diagnoses related to infant growth and development and associated parental concerns.

4. Identify outcomes to promote optimal infant growth and development and health.

5. Plan nursing care to meet the infant's growth and development needs.

6. Implement nursing care related to normal growth and development of the infant.

7. Evaluate outcomes for achievement of optimal growth and development and effectiveness of care.

8. Identify National Health Goals related to infant growth and development that nurses can be instrumental in helping the nation achieve.

9. Identify areas related to nursing care of the infant that could benefit from additional nursing research or application of evidence-based practice.

10. Use critical thinking to analyze methods of care for the infant to be certain care is family-centered.

11. Integrate knowledge of infant growth and development with nursing process to achieve quality maternal and child health nursing care.

KEY TERMS

baby-bottle syndrome
binocular vision
coordination of secondary schema
deciduous teeth
eighth-month anxiety
extrusion reflex
fine motor development
gross motor development
hand regard
Landau reflex
natal teeth
neck-righting reflex

neonatal teeth
object permanence
parachute reaction
pincer grasp
prehensile ability
primary circular reaction
seborrhea
secondary circular reaction
social smile
thumb opposition
ventral suspension

■ Section One:
Identification of Key Terms and Concepts

Match the fine motor skills listed in Part A with the appropriate age of onset found in Part B. Place the letter corresponding to the answer in the space provided. (Letters may be used more than once, but there is only one answer for each number.)

PART A

1. _____ Brings hands together and pulls

2. _____ Has pincer grasp and points

3. _____ Transfers toys from hand to hand

4. _____ Ineffective grasping disappears

5. _____ Stranger anxiety

6. _____ Supports nearly his or her full weight while standing

7. _____ Enjoys putting things in and taking things out of containers

8. _____ Shows displeasure

9. _____ Laughs

PART B

A. 3 months

B. 4 months

C. 6 months

D. 7 months

E. 8 months

F. 10 months

G. 12 months

■ Section Two:
Short Answer and Completion Exercises

Complete the following short answer exercises.

1. State four benefits derived from well-child follow-up visits.

   _____   _____

   _____   _____

2. At what age does an infant's immune system becomes functional? _____

3. The first tooth eruption is expected at what age? _____

4. What is the most serious complication for infants with supernumerary teeth?

   _____

5. At what age should an infant begin to demonstrate the ability to sit without support? _____

6. Identify the four body positions from which to assess gross motor development in an infant.

   _____   _____

   _____   _____

7. List three ways parents can childproof their homes.

   _____   _____

   _____

8. Identify two benefits to the growth and development of infants that may be promoted when bathing the infant.

   _____   _____

9. How can parents provide tooth and oral care for their infants?

10. State three ways to prevent diaper dermatitis.

    _____   _____

    _____

11. State three common causes of constipation.

    _____   _____

    _____

12. What are three factors that should be assessed when an infant is experiencing diarrhea?

    _____   _____

    _____

■ Section Three:
Critical Thinking for Application of Essential Concepts

PART 1

Circle the letter corresponding to the appropriate answer.

1. During a routine well-child visit the nurse should educate the parents regarding

   A. the infant's need for meat by 4 months of age.

   B. expected growth and development patterns.

   C. specific yearly milestones the child must meet.

   D. the signs and symptoms of failure to thrive.

2. According to Erikson's theory of emotional development, infants will develop a sense of trust when

   A. they can identify their mother and father.

   B. they feel a sense of belonging, accepted as part of the family.

   C. they can predict what is coming and needs are consistently met.

   D. nutritional and hygiene needs are provided on a daily basis.

3. Keeping in mind the leading cause of accidents in infants, the nurse should advise parents to

   A. buy clothes for the infant with buttons rather than snaps.

   B. check all toys for small removable parts.

   C. provide round, cylinder-type toys.

   D. avoid finger foods before the age of 15 months.

4. Since falls are a common cause of injury to infants, parents should be advised to

   A. avoid using pillows around the infant placed on a bed.

   B. use an infant seat when placing the infant on a table top.

   C. use blankets around the infant on a couch.

   D. place protective gates at the top and bottom of stairs.

5. Palliative measures aimed at relieving colic should include

   A. placing a warm heating pad on the abdomen.

   B. diluting the formula to a weaker strength.

   C. administering simethicone at 30-minute intervals.

   D. sitting the infant upright for a half-hour after feedings.

6. Alice is 4 months of age. Her mother is singing to her. Why type of response should be expected of Alice?

   A. Imitating the sounds

   B. Smiling, cooing, and gurgling

   C. Saying "da-da"

   D. Watching her mother's face without making a sound

7. Patrick is 10 months old. What type of play activity is appropriate for his expected level of development?

   A. Rolling a ball

   B. Shaking a rattle

   C. Winding up a toy

   D. Playing patty-cake

8. At what age should an infant begin to locate an object hidden under a blanket?

   A. 6 months

   B. 8 months

   C. 10 months

   D. 12 months

9. When assessing the visual ability of a 7-month-old boy, the nurse should

   A. attempt to place a familiar object in the infant's hand and observe his response.

   B. use a brightly colored object and check the infant's ability to follow the object.

   C. use a mirror to observe the infant's response to his image.

   D. observe the infant's ability to follow hand motions.

10. Tracey, a 6-month-old, is undergoing a hearing assessment. Would you expect her to be able to locate sounds made at a distance over her head?

    A. Yes

    B. No

11. Most infants should be expected to sleep

    A. 10 to 12 hours per night, with one or more naps.

    B. 14 to 16 hours per night, with one nap.

    C. an average of 18 to 20 hours each day.

    D. at 4-hour intervals and throughout the night

12. What type of device would enhance the development of an 8-month-old infant through play activity?

    A. Stroller

    B. Floor mat

    C. Crib

    D. Play pen

13. A major developmental task for the family of an infant girl should be

    A. interpreting her cues to decipher her needs.

    B. gaining her autonomy and freedom to express herself.

    C. providing an environment for learning new skills.

    D. allowing her to take initiative and respond to her environment.

14. An 8-month-old infant who loves to suck her thumb visits the clinic. Her mother is very worried that this habit will cause permanent dental problems. What should the nurse advise the mother to do?

   A. Wrap her thumb with adhesive tape.

   B. Distract her with toys.

   C. Ignore this behavior.

   D. Remove her thumb from her mouth as often as possible.

15. Parents report their infant frequently wakes up from a sound sleep. What should the nurse advise the parents to do to help her sleep through the night?

   A. When the infant awakens, wait a while and she will fall back to sleep.

   B. Go to her immediately when she awakens and comfort her back to sleep.

   C. Soothe her back to sleep with her favorite toy and soft music.

   D. Pick her up and rock her back to sleep.

PART 2: CASE STUDY

Stephen is a 5-month-old infant visiting the well-child clinic for his second series of immunizations.

1. Stephen weighed 7 lb and was 20 inches long at birth. Based on normal growth and development parameters, what should his weight be at this visit?

2. List a normal set of vital signs that may be assessed from Stephen.

3. On what physiologic principle might the physician prescribe a vitamin with iron?

4. Stephen's mother is eager to feed him solid foods and asks the nurse if it would be recommended. What response would the nurse give? Why?

■ Section Four: Inquiry and Exploration

PART 1: CRITICAL INQUIRY EXERCISES

1. Formulate a nursing care plan for the following case scenario: David, a 7-month-old infant, is experiencing diarrhea. His weight was 18 lb before the diarrhea; now it is 16 lb. His anterior fontanel is slightly sunken, mucous membranes are dry, urine output is diminished, and the specific gravity is 1.035.

2. Contrast the developmental milestones occurring during infancy relating to fine and gross motor skills and physiologic and cognitive development.

PART 2: CRITICAL EXPLORATION EXERCISES

Assess two infants of the same chronologic age, but one born at term and one born 2 to 3 months prematurely. Make an assessment of the developmental behaviors that are seen in the adjusted chronologic age groups for these infants. Comparatively evaluate the infants' performances. What principles of growth and development should be researched for this exercise?

CHAPTER 29

The Family With a Toddler

CHAPTER OVERVIEW

This chapter explores the patterns of normal growth and development of the toddler. The developmental accomplishments related to fine and gross motor skills and language skills are presented. Anticipatory guidance with a reference to making the toddler's environment safe is also addressed. The case study provides the student with the opportunity to provide teaching for the parents of a toddler through a teaching plan for health promotion.

LEARNING OBJECTIVES

After mastering the contents of this chapter, you should be able to:

1. Describe normal growth and development of the toddler period as well as common parental concerns.

2. Assess a toddler for normal growth and development milestones.

3. Formulate nursing diagnoses related to toddler growth and development or parental concerns regarding development.

4. Identify expected outcomes for nursing care of the toddler.

5. Plan nursing care to meet the toddler's growth and development needs, such as anticipatory guidance to prevent problems such as sleep disturbances, temper tantrums, or inappropriate toilet training practices.

6. Implement nursing care to promote normal growth and development of the toddler, such as discussing toddler developmental milestones with parents.

7. Evaluate goal outcomes established for care to be certain nursing goals associated with growth and development have been achieved.

8. Identify National Health Goals related to the toddler age group that nurses can be instrumental in helping the nation to achieve.

9. Identify areas related to care of the toddler that could benefit from additional nursing research or application of evidence-based practice.

10. Use critical thinking to analyze methods of care for the toddler to be certain care is family-centered.

11. Integrate knowledge of toddler growth and development with nursing process to achieve quality maternal and child health nursing care.

KEY TERMS

assimilation
autonomy
deferred imitation
discipline
lordosis

parallel play
preoperational thought
punishment
tertiary circular reaction stage

■ Section One:
Identification of Key Terms and Concepts

Match the terms in Part A with a definition or related statement from Part B. Place the letter corresponding to the answer in the space provided.

PART A

1. _____ Deferred imitation

2. _____ Negativism

3. _____ Separation anxiety

4. _____ Lordosis

5. _____ Discipline

6. _____ Preoperational thought

PART B

A. Universal fear that begins at about 6 months of age and persists thro ughout the preschool period

B. Remembering an action to mimic at a later time

C. A forward curve of the spine at the sacral area

D. A positive stage in toddler development; the toddler sees himself or herself as a separate individual with separate needs

E. Major period of cognitive development that usually occurs at the end of the toddler period

F. Setting rules to teach children what is expected of them

■ Section Two:
Short Answer and Completion Exercises

Describe the gross motor, language, and play developmental milestones that are accomplished at ages 15, 24, and 30 months.

■ Section Three: Critical Thinking for Application of Essential Concepts

PART 1

Circle the letter corresponding to the appropriate answer.

1. The child's universal language is
   A. behavior.
   B. crying.
   C. touching.
   D. play.

2. Which of the following describes the type of play observed with toddlers?
   A. Solitary
   B. Parallel
   C. Competitive
   D. Fantasy

3. A major source for reducing the incidence of lead poisoning is
   A. parent education.
   B. early detection.
   C. family planning.
   D. chelating therapy.

4. All of the following may be symptoms of a child experiencing lead poisoning except
   A. irritability.
   B. cardiomegaly.
   C. headaches.
   D. abdominal pain.

5. Which of the following may represent an emotional stress from hospitalization usually experienced by the toddler?
   A. Loss of control
   B. Fear of bodily injury
   C. Fear of death
   D. Separation anxiety

6. When communicating with a toddler who is subject to feelings of separation anxiety, it is recommended that you
   A. call him by name as you greet him.
   B. introduce yourself by first name, then ask his name.
   C. talk softly and kneel in front of or beside him
   D. state clearly that you are his nurse.

PART 2

Determine if the following nursing interventions are appropriate or inappropriate.
Indicate your answer by placing an "A" or an "I" in the space provided.

1. _____ Leaving toddlers alone in the tub for a brief moment while bathing them

2. _____ Offering high-protein snacks rather than high-carbohydrate snacks

3. _____ Placing a gate on the door to a toddler's room

4. _____ Informing parents that sleep times will be shorter for toddlers than for infants

5. _____ Offering a toddler something pleasurable in the middle of a temper tantrum to stop the tantrum

6. _____ Assisting the child in putting his clothes on correctly to develop neatness

7. _____ Placing medicines on shelves at least 4 feet high to be out of a child's reach

8. _____ Encouraging parents to buy arch-supportive shoes

9. _____ Attempting to potty-train a child who is about 2 years of age

10. _____ Choosing a potty-chair that sits on the commode

PART 3: CASE STUDY

Mr. and Mrs. Stargell and their 18-month-old son, Cody, are being seen today in the pediatrician's office where you are a nurse for a follow-up visit. The night before, Mr. Stargell discovered that Cody had tumbled down the stairs. The Stargells called the emergency room at a local children's hospital; they were instructed to bring Cody to the ER immediately. Cody was given a thorough examination and was treated for a small laceration to the head and a severely sprained arm. He was discharged in stable condition from the ER with instructions to see the pediatrician the following morning.

1. What information regarding toddler safety should you include in your plan to teach health promotion to Cody's parents?

2. You begin your assessment of Cody with a careful health history. What is the rationale for taking this health history?

3. Explain how information from a health history will help you develop a teaching plan for Cody's parents.

■ Section Four: Inquiry and Exploration

PART 1: CRITICAL INQUIRY EXERCISES

1. Formulate a nursing care plan that will focus on setting safety guidelines for an 18-month-old child in the home environment.

2. List outcome criteria that might be established before the parents leave the pediatrician's office.

PART 2: CRITICAL EXPLORATION EXERCISES

1. Visit a day-care setting and observe a group of toddlers during a free play period for 30 minutes or more. Select one toddler from the group and describe how he or she plays among the group members.

2. Visit the Red Cross center in your community and obtain the name and address of an agency that will furnish literature to institutions or families on poison prevention and child safety. Write for the literature and ask your instructor for assistance to distribute the materials to the parents of the children at your pediatric clinical site.

CHAPTER 30

The Family With a Preschooler

CHAPTER OVERVIEW

Preschool-age children demonstrate the desire to care for themselves through daily activities. They insist on dressing themselves and often resist assistance from parents. The nurse should include the need for parent education related to these behaviors when planning nursing care. This chapter discusses the developmental tasks and anticipatory guidance for children in this age group. The case study provides a learning opportunity for sex education during the preschool years.

LEARNING OBJECTIVES

After mastering the contents of this chapter, you should be able to:

1. Describe normal growth and development as well as common parental concerns of the preschool period.

2. Assess a preschooler for normal growth and developmental milestones.

3. Formulate nursing diagnoses related to preschool growth and development and common parental concerns.

4. Identify expected outcomes for nursing care of the toddler.

5. Plan nursing care to meet the preschooler's growth and development needs, such as planning age-appropriate play activities.

6. Implement nursing care related to normal growth and development of the preschooler, such as preparing a preschooler for an invasive procedure.

7. Evaluate outcome criteria established for care to be certain normal growth and development goals have been achieved.

8. Identify National Health Goals related to the preschool period that nurses can be instrumental in helping the nation to achieve.

9. Identify areas related to care of the preschool-age child that could benefit from additional nursing research or application of evidence-based practice.

10. Use critical thinking to analyze additional ways in which growth and developmental problems of the preschool child can be prevented and care can be family-centered.

11. Integrate knowledge of preschool growth and development with nursing process to achieve quality maternal and child health nursing care.

KEY TERMS

broken fluency	endomorphic body build
bruxism	genu valgus
conservation	intuitional thought
ectomorphic body build	Oedipus complex
Electra complex	secondary stuttering

■ Section One:
Identification of Key Terms and Concepts

Match the terms in Part A with a definition or related statement from Part B. Place the letter corresponding to the answer in the space provided.

PART A

1. _____ Initiative versus guilt

2. _____ Play

3. _____ Regression

4. _____ Broken fluency

5. _____ Intuitional thought

PART B

A. Reverting to behaviors practiced in earlier years

B. Repetition and prolongation of sounds

C. Preschoolers engaged in this are guided by their imaginations

D. Stage of cognitive development in which preschoolers lack the insight to view themselves as others see them and think of themselves as always right

E. A child who has achieved this task knows that learning about new things is fun and is not afraid to try a new task

■ Section Two:
Short Answer and Completion Exercises

PART 1

Define the following terms.

1. Endomorphic _____

2. Ectomorphic _____

3. Genu valgus _____

4. Bruxism _____

PART 2

Complete the following short answer exercises.

1. Describe the Oedipus and Electra complexes.

2. Explain how the preschooler's inability to understand the law of conservation may affect your ability to care for him or her.

3. What are some therapeutic methods that can be practiced by the nurse and family to alleviate the preschooler's fear of the dark?

4. Identify four basic rules recommended to resolve secondary stuttering.

■ Section Three: Critical Thinking for Application of Essential Concepts

PART 1

Circle the letter corresponding to the appropriate answer.

1. Which of the following types of play is primarily demonstrated by preschoolers?
    A. Parallel
    B. Imaginary
    C. Solitary
    D. Cooperative

2. If the preschooler is hospitalized, which of the following is likely to describe his or her feelings?
    A. Frustrated by the need to alter his or her rituals
    B. Depressed and angry
    C. Fearful of losing his or her self-esteem
    D. Restricted and restrained from mobilization

3. What is the appropriate action to lessen the feelings of rivalry among siblings?
   A. Punish for unacceptable behavior.
   B. Separate siblings and give individual attention separately.
   C. Interact with younger and older siblings together.
   D. Allow the older sibling to practice adult roles to comfort him or her.

4. A preschooler appropriately explores his body by
   A. dressing up in parents' clothing.
   B. masturbating.
   C. inflicting harm.
   D. comparing his body parts with playmates.

5. Which of the following is an appropriate activity for the preschooler?
   A. Cutting paper dolls
   B. Checkers
   C. "London Bridge"
   D. Dart board game

PART 2

Determine if the following nursing interventions are appropriate or inappropriate. Indicate your answer by placing an "A" or an "I" in the space provided.

1. _____ Encourage the preschooler to speak during the health examination.

2. _____ Assess weight and height or standard growth chart at each health visit.

3. _____ Include head circumference on each physical examination.

4. _____ Encourage constructive play.

5. _____ Provide a helmet for bicycle riding.

6. _____ Use a plastic visor while taking a bath.

7. _____ Turn the water heater to 110° to 120°F.

8. _____ Allow the preschooler to floss his or her teeth at least once a day.

9. _____ Burn a dim light in the child's room at night.

10. _____ Provide the preschooler with a private space for his or her belongings that is not to be shared.

PART 3: CASE STUDY

Mrs. Bell and her two children, Amy (age 8) and Bryan (age 4), are visiting the health center today for a well-child appointment. Mrs. Bell is 6 months pregnant. After the physician's visit, Mrs. Bell asks if she could speak with you for a few moments about Bryan. She explains that she is very concerned about Bryan's fixation on his genitals. Mrs. Bell began to notice this behavior about 2 weeks after she enrolled him in a day-care center. She says that he masturbates often and seems to have forgotten what the family has taught him about his "private parts."

1. What is the developmental theory that would suggest why Bryan has started to demonstrate this behavior?

2. What guidelines would you use to advise Mrs. Bell regarding Bryan's masturbating in public?

3. What basic rule concerning sex education should you be sure to mention to help protect Bryan from sexual abuse?

4. Outline a teaching plan to help the mother explain pregnancy and the arrival of a new baby.

■ Section Four: Inquiry and Exploration

PART 1: CRITICAL INQUIRY EXERCISES

1. Contrast the developmental milestones across the life span of the 3-, 4-, and 5-year-old.

2. Prepare a teaching plan for the parent and preschooler about developing safety measures in the home.

PART 2: CRITICAL EXPLORATION EXERCISES

1. Visit a kindergarten and talk with a preschool child near the end of the day. Ask the child to tell you what happened during the day. Assess the child's language development, understand how the term "egocentrism" applies to the preschooler, and identify if the child is accomplishing the developmental tasks of that age group.

2. Visit a preschool child who is hospitalized for an elective surgery. Talk to the child before the surgery. Obtain three or four pictures depicting a pediatric hospital area, including the patient's room and the operating room. Do not include any pictures suggestive of invasive procedures or treatment. Show these pictures to the preschooler and ask him or her to make up a story about the pictures. Record the story as the preschooler talks to you. Identify the statements indicating fear and stress. Notice in the story how the child's ability to fantasize allows him or her to stretch the imagination to include even mutilation, although the pictures do not suggest aggressive or invasive subjects.

CHAPTER 31

The Family With a School-Age Child

CHAPTER OVERVIEW

The school-age years (ages 6 to 12) represent a time of slow physical growth, but cognitive and developmental growth is rapid. When caring for this age group, it is important to stress the physical growth and accomplishment of emotional, cognitive, and moral developmental tasks. The school-age period is the time the child becomes independent and begins to separate from the family for long periods of time. The nurse should know the principles of development related to this age group to promote developmental needs and safety. This chapter contains exercises that help the student in learning developmental tasks and in assisting the family of a school-age child by providing anticipatory guidance. The case study emphasizes the principles of school-age growth and development.

LEARNING OBJECTIVES

After mastering the contents of this chapter, you should be able to:

1. Describe the normal growth and development pattern and common parental concerns of the school-age period.

2. Assess a school-age child for normal growth and development milestones.

3. Formulate nursing diagnoses for the family of a school-age child.

4. Identify expected outcomes based on health assessment findings.

5. Plan anticipatory guidance to prevent problems of growth and development in the school-age child (e.g., teaching about normal puberty).

6. Implement nursing care to help achieve normal growth and development of the school-age child, such as counseling parents about helping their child adjust to a new school.

7. Evaluate outcome criteria to be certain that goals of care have been achieved.

8. Identify National Health Goals related to the school-age child that nurses can be instrumental in helping the nation achieve.

9. Identify areas related to care of school-age children that could benefit from additional nursing research or application of evidence-based practice.

10. Use critical thinking to analyze ways in which the care of the school-age child can be more family-centered.

11. Integrate knowledge of school-age growth and development with the nursing process to achieve quality maternal and child health nursing care.

KEY TERMS

accommodation   inclusion
caries   latchkey child
class inclusion   malocclusion
conservation   nocturnal emissions
decenter   preconventional reasoning

▪ Section One:
Identification of Key Terms and Concepts

Match the chronologic school age in Part A with the physical or psychosocial development in Part B. Place the letter corresponding to the answer in the space provided.

PART A

1. _____ Age 6

2. _____ Age 7

3. _____ Age 8

4. _____ Age 9

5. _____ Age 10

6. _____ Age 11

7. _____ Age 12

PART B

A. Best friends are important; enjoys whispering and giggling

B. Teacher becomes authority figure

C. Social and cooperative

D. Central incisors erupt (youngest age)

E. Coordination improves (youngest age)

F. Clubs are formed, all boys or all girls

G. Insecure with members of opposite sex

▪ Section Two:
Short Answer and Completion Exercises

PART 1

Complete the following fill-in-the-blank exercises.

1. The androgen hormone stimulates the growth of the _____ and

   _____ in girls, and the _____ and _____ in males.

2. Talent for music or art becomes evident and children respond well by age

   _____.

PART 2

Complete the following short answer exercises.

1. List the gonadotropic hormones and give the function of each.

2. Compare and contrast the accomplishment or failure of the developmental task industry versus inferiority.

3. Describe the characteristics of the following forms of cognitive development:

   Decenter

   Accommodation

   Conservation

   Class inclusion

4. What advice would you give parents to improve or increase their child's interest in reading?

5. Define school phobia. Discuss why this occurs and give ways to help the family cope with and resolve these fears.

PART 3

Describe measures that can be taken to avoid accidents with the school-age child.

1. Drowning

2. Motor vehicle accident

3. Sports injuries

4. Community

5. Firearms

▪ Section Three:
Critical Thinking for Application of Essential Concepts

PART 1

Circle the letter corresponding to the appropriate answer.

1. Sex education should be introduced at
   A. high school.
   B. junior high school.
   C. middle school.
   D. grade/elementary school.

2. The gross motor development of a 6-year-old will allow her to
   A. jump, tumble, skip, stumble, and hop endlessly.
   B. play hopscotch and skip rope well.
   C. ride a bicycle and play hopscotch.
   D. jump, tumble, and skip rope well.

3. Peer relationships are important to the school-age child. Which of the following is a characteristic of the 9-year-old?

   A. Boys and girls love to play together.

   B. Activities are very complete.

   C. Boys and girls begin to have social interactions.

   D. Loyalty and affiliation are directed to a group of same-sex peers.

4. Which of the following behaviors denotes stress when displayed by the 6- or 7-year-old child?

   A. Tics

   B. Crying

   C. Bed-wetting

   D. Swearing

5. Which of the following is correct regarding physical maturation before puberty?

   A. Boys are usually taller than girls.

   B. Girls are usually taller than boys.

PART 2: CASE STUDY

Mrs. Elway brings her daughter Clois, age 11, to the well-child care center for an annual check-up. The nurse obtains the history and begins the assessment. Clois's vital signs are within normal limits: temperature 98.6°F, pulse 75, respirations 26, blood pressure 110/58. Mrs. Elway tells the nurse she is concerned about Clois's sudden outbreaks of perspiration; although the episodes are not frequent, they don't seem to correlate with environmental temperatures.

1. What anticipatory guidance should the nurse give to Mrs. Elway regarding breast development and vaginal secretion?

2. Clois wants to play soccer at school; Mrs. Elway asks the nurse if she thinks this would be a good idea. What principles regarding structured activities should the nurse call upon to formulate a response?

▪ Section Four: Inquiry and Exploration

PART 1: CRITICAL INQUIRY EXERCISES

1. Develop a teaching plan for parents to explain the physical growth related to sexuality occurring during the school-age years.

2. Create a set of key points to discuss when providing anticipatory guidance for parents on detection of recreational drug use.

PART 2: CRITICAL EXPLORATION EXERCISES

1. Observe students in an elementary school classroom. Record the behaviors of the teacher that may be considered positive and valuable to the children's transition to the school environment.

2. Observe several students for gross and fine motor development. Compare the findings to the expected motor development for that chronologic age group.

3. Visit a school during a recess period and observe the behaviors of children that are active with the following types of play: (a) group, (b) cooperative, (c) grouping, (d) same gender, and (e) consisting of rules.

The Family With an Adolescent

CHAPTER OVERVIEW

Chapter 32 provides an overview of adolescent growth and development, nursing care related to health promotion, and the management of illness in the adolescent. The physiologic and psychological needs of the adolescent and common health concerns encountered during adolescence are reviewed. The use of the nursing process to plan and provide appropriate health care for the adolescent and his or her family is explored.

LEARNING OBJECTIVES

After mastering the contents of this chapter, you should be able to:

1. Describe the normal growth and development pattern and common parental concerns of the adolescent period.

2. Assess adolescents for normal growth and development milestones.

3. Formulate nursing diagnoses for the family of an adolescent.

4. Identify expected outcomes based on health assessment findings.

5. Plan nursing care related to growth and development concerns of the adolescent, such as planning health teaching necessary to accept pubertal changes.

6. Implement nursing care related to growth and development or special needs of the adolescent, such as organizing a discussion group on ways to prevent drug abuse.

7. Evaluate expected outcomes to be certain that nursing care was comprehensive.

8. Identify National Health Goals related to the adolescent that nurses could be instrumental in helping the nation to achieve.

9. Identify areas related to care of adolescents that could benefit from additional nursing research or application of evidence-based practice.

10. Use critical thinking to analyze ways in which care of the adolescent could be more family-centered.

11. Integrate knowledge of adolescent growth and development with nursing process to achieve quality maternal and child health nursing care.

KEY TERMS

adolescence
comedones
formal operations
glycogen loading
identity

puberty
role confusion
stalking
substance abuse

■ Section One:
Identification of Key Terms and Concepts

Match the terms in Part A with a definition or related statement from Part B. Place the letter corresponding to the answer in the space provided.

PART A

1. _____ Adolescence

2. _____ Cognitive development

3. _____ Empathy

4. _____ Intimacy

5. _____ Substance abuse

6. _____ Puberty

7. _____ Pustular acne

8. _____ Runaway

9. _____ Suicide

10. _____ Secondary sex characteristics

PART B

A. The physiologic period between the beginning of puberty and the cessation of bodily growth

B. Use of chemicals to improve the mental state

C. Deliberate self-injury with the intent to end one's life

D. Body hair configuration and breast growth; aid in distinguishing males from females, but play no part in reproduction

E. Feeling for another by projecting one's self into the other person's situation

F. Involves developing a sense of compassion or concern for others

G. The stage at which the individual first becomes capable of sexual reproduction

H. Adolescent between 10 and 17 years old who is absent from home at least overnight without permission of parent or guardian

I. Often treated with systemic antibiotics

J. Involves the ability to think in abstract terms and use the scientific method

■ Section Two:
Short Answer and Completion Exercises

PART 1

Complete the following fill-in-the-blank exercises.

1. One major dilemma encountered by adolescents that leads to many growth and development concerns is that they are _____ in some respects but still _____ in others.

2. Females generally stop growing within _____ years from menarche.

3. Adolescents will experience a slight _____ in pulse rate and a slight _____ in blood pressure as they move toward adulthood.

4. Early adolescence generally occurs between the ages of _____ and ____ years; middle adolescence occurs between _____ and ____ years; and late adolescence occurs between _____ and _____ years.

5. Cognitive development over the adolescent years involves the stage of _____ _____ , which begins at age _____ or _____ .

6. The goal of therapy for acne treatment is to decrease _____ _____ , prevent _____ , and control _____ _____ .

7. As many as 90% of high school seniors report having used _____ .

PART 2

Complete the following short answer exercises.

1. Discuss two reasons the nurse should obtain an adolescent's health history in private, separately from his or her parents.

   _____   _____

2. List three common factors (primary assessment areas) that explain why adolescents may suffer fatigue.

   _____   _____

   _____

3. What major task must the adolescent achieve in each of the following developmental areas: sense of intimacy, emancipation from parents, and value system?

4. State two ways nurses can be instrumental in helping to achieve National Health Goals related to adolescent health.

   _____   _____

5. Describe the common social behaviors manifested by adolescents at ages 13, 14, 15, 16, and 17.

6. Identify 7 of the 14 danger signs for adolescent suicide.

   _____   _____

   _____   _____

   _____   _____

   _____

■ Section Three: Critical Thinking for Application of Essential Concepts

PART 1

Circle the letter corresponding to the appropriate answer.

1. Because of changes occurring in the sebaceous glands and sweat glands of adolescents, the nurse would include which of the following in health care teaching?

   A. Increased hygiene requirements to reduce body odor and acne

   B. Information regarding the need for increased fat-soluble vitamins

   C. Instructions regarding medications for inadequate sweat production

   D. Exercises that will minimize the production of sweat

2. When planning a teaching strategy for an adolescent, the nurse should do which of the following?

   A. Give information about how the teen can manage the specific problems he or she identifies.

   B. Maintain an air of authority by providing explanations for care procedures to parents only.

   C. Provide information related to long-term health needs, since adolescents respond best to long-range planning.

   D. Teach the parents first, since they will be better able to teach the teen.

3. At his physical, Bob, 14 years old, tells the nurse he is "a short, clumsy klutz." The nurse should respond in which of the following ways?

   A. Discuss with Bob the fact that his clumsiness is probably a sign of an easily curable disease.

   B. Instruct Bob in methods of relieving clumsiness through muscle exercises and improving nutrition.

   C. Explain to Bob that adolescent boys are usually taller than adolescent girls, so he should be examined.

   D. Inform Bob that he will probably grow taller over the next 4 to 6 years and become more coordinated.

4. The mother of Sheila, age 13, reports that Sheila "talks for hours to her girl-friends, and spends most of her waking hours with girls." The nurse could reassure Sheila's mother by explaining which of the following?

   A. If Sheila spends less time on the phone during the next 2 years, she will mature normally.

   B. Sheila is probably talking to boys when her parents aren't around.

   C. Talking on the phone and spending time with girlfriends is normal for a girl of Sheila's age.

   D. There is no current threat of homosexuality due to Sheila's young age.

5. Marla is 15 years old. Marla's mother tells the nurse she fears that her daughter will get into serious trouble soon because she is always "going for a walk or sitting outside somewhere." The nurse should respond in which of the following ways to this information?

   A. Encourage Marla's mother to follow her to determine why Marla is being so distant.

   B. Inform the mother that Marla is probably all right and is seeking the privacy she needs.

   C. Schedule Marla for a blood and urine drug screening immediately.

   D. Tell Marla's mother to call a psychologist to help her deal with the stress of adolescence.

6. Which of the following would be a positive sign of identity formation in a client in late adolescence?

   A. Obtaining a job and saving money

   B. Continuous dieting

   C. Getting pregnant and having a baby

   D. Living with parents

7. Daryl, age 17, states he shouldn't have sex and get girls pregnant "mostly because my parents would be really mad." Daryl's response may indicate a lack of development in which of the following areas?

   A. Cognitive development

   B. Moral development

   C. Physiologic development

   D. Religious development

8. A realistic outcome criterion related to an adolescent with a history of experimentation with marijuana would be that the adolescent would do which of the following?

A. Stop using drugs immediately without assistance.

B. Discuss ways to enjoy life without drugs.

C. Use only marijuana, with no additional drug use.

D. Smoke marijuana in moderation.

9. Which of the following would be a realistic outcome criterion related to an adolescent with a medical condition requiring a special diet?

A. The adolescent with diabetes will eat no sweet, sugary foods.

B. The adolescent with hypertension will not eat potato chips.

C. The adolescent with fatigue will choose preferred foods that contain a high vitamin and mineral content.

D. The adolescent with acne will discuss the need for foods high in lipids to replace the deficient body supply.

10. Anna, age 17, has been identified as a suicide risk. The nurse should watch her carefully and during discharge teaching discuss the need for the family to watch her particularly closely

A. before the beginning of the school year.

B. between noon and 3 p.m.

C. during her menstrual period.

D. late at night.

PART 2

Determine if the following nursing interventions for adolescent abuse of the specified drug are appropriate or inappropriate. Indicate your answer by placing an "A" or an "I" in the space provided.

1. _____ Alcohol: Investigate the presence of alcohol abuse by parents or other close family members.

2. _____ Amphetamines: Monitor for symptoms such as aggressive and demanding behavior and paranoia.

3. _____ Anabolic steroids: Instruct athletes that these drugs cause fatigue and depression, which will lead to weight gain.

4. _____ Barbiturates: Allow the suicide-prone adolescent the control of managing oral administration alone, since these are generally harmless drugs.

5. _____ Cigarettes: Have a nurse who smokes discuss with the teen the evils and problems caused by smoking as one who knows the problems personally.

6. _____ Cocaine/crack: Educate adolescents on the potential for immediate death even with the first use.

7. _____ LSD/PCP: Inform teens that this drug can cause brain damage and dangerous flashbacks.

8. _____ Marijuana: Emphasize that short-term use can cause pulmonary problems, although low but consistent use over several years has shown no harmful effects.

9. ____ Opiates: Discuss the potential for exposure to the AIDS virus when shared needles are used.

10. ____ All drugs: Emphasize the fact that there are no "good" drugs, and that marijuana can lead to more dangerous drugs.

PART 3: CASE STUDY

Angelique Rodriguez, age 14, was referred to you, the school nurse, by her guidance counselor. Angelique's grades have dropped from A's to low C's over the past two semesters, and she has become aggressive and refuses to talk to the teachers or counselors. The counselor suspects drugs, pregnancy, or depression but doesn't know how to help Angelique.

1. What would three of your first actions be when approaching Angelique?

2. What permissions would you need from Angelique and her parents, and what actions could you take without contacting her parents?

3. If Angelique admitted depression and drug abuse, what initial steps would you take to get help for her?

■ Section Four:
Inquiry and Exploration

PART 1: CRITICAL INQUIRY EXERCISES

1. Prepare a teaching plan for an adolescent group that addresses methods for maintaining adequate nutrition, rest, and exercise.

2. How could the usual social behaviors noted in adolescents ages 13 through 17 contribute to problems or concerns that may be experienced by the adolescent and his or her family?

PART 2: CRITICAL EXPLORATION EXERCISES

Attend a group session at an adolescent drug rehabilitation center (either in person or via two-way mirror). Note common themes related to why adolescents use drugs.

CHAPTER 33

Child Health Assessment

CHAPTER OVERVIEW

This chapter offers an in-depth discussion of the nursing techniques used in child health assessment. Interviewing skills and procedures for performing physical and developmental assessments are described. Nursing interventions aimed at reducing the child's anxiety during assessment procedures are given. Normal growth and development parameters and health deviations are explained for each component of the health assessment. A case study is presented to help the student study the principles used in conducting an abdominal assessment.

LEARNING OBJECTIVES

After mastering the contents of this chapter, you should be able to:

1. State the purposes for health assessment in children of all ages.

2. Assess a child and family by health interview, physical examination, and development screening.

3. Use the nursing process to determine and address nursing diagnoses based on health assessment findings.

4. Identify National Health Goals related to health assessment of children that nurses can be instrumental in helping the nation achieve.

5. Identify areas related to health assessment of children that could benefit from additional nursing research.

6. Use critical thinking to analyze ways that health assessment skills can be incorporated into nursing care procedures.

7. Synthesize the nursing process with knowledge of health assessment to achieve quality maternal and child health nursing care.

KEY TERMS

audiogram	general appearance	physiologic splitting
auscultation	geographic tongue	point of maximum impulse
bruit	gingivae	ptosis
chief concern	hordeolum	retractions
cognitive learning	hydrocele	review of systems
conjunctivitis	hypospadias	sinus arrhythmia
deep tendon reflexes	inspection	strabismus
diaphragmatic excursion	intelligence	superficial reflexes
epispadias	intercostal spaces	temperament
esotropia	kwashiorkor	tinea capitis
exotropia	palpation	turgor
fasciculations	percussion	varicocele

■ Section One: Identification of Key Terms and Concepts

PART 1

Identify the following types of interview questions. Place the letter corresponding to the answer in the space provided.

Types of Question
P - 942/943

PART A

1. __C__ "Tell me about Tommy's health."

2. __D__ "Jamie doesn't like to sleep in her crib, does she?"

3. __A__ "When did Bobby start walking?"

4. __B__ "Is Alice allergic to wheat and oats?"

5. __D__ "Why does Greg hate taking his medication?"

PART B

A. Open-ended question

B. Compound question

C. Expansive question

D. Leading question

PART 2

Match the following child health problems with the correct signs and symptoms that may be noted on the extremities. Place the letter corresponding to the answer in the space provided.

PART A

1. __B__ Iron deficiency anemia B

2. __C__ Cyanosis C

3. _____ Endocarditis D

4. _____ Chromosomal abnormalities A

PART B

A. Simian crease

B. Concave nails

C. Clubbed fingers

D. Linear hemorrhages under the nails

■ Section Two: Short Answer and Completion Exercises

PART 1

Complete the following fill-in-the-blank exercises.

1. The mobility of the eardrum (tympanic membrane) can be tested by injecting _____ into the ear canal.

2. _____ is a rough-appearing tongue surface that accompanies general symptoms of illness such as fever.

3. Sinus arrhythmias are considered a normal phenomenon in children of _____ age. They are characterized by a marked heart rate increase on _____ and a marked heart rate decrease on _____.

PART 2

Complete the following short answer exercises.

1. List and explain the eight categories for data gathering in performing the initial health assessment for the child and family.

   Health History   _____
   demographic   _____
   chief concern   _____
   _____   _____

2. What are the height and weight deviations that indicate failure to thrive syndrome in an infant?

3. Name two tests used to detect strabismus.

   _____   _____

4. Describe the assessment technique used to detect choanal atresia.

5. Name three prominent features of chronic serous otitis media.

   _____   _____
   _____

6. List five high-risk conditions that are associated with hearing impairment in children.

_____   _____

_____   _____

_____

■ Section Three:
Critical Thinking for Application of Essential Concepts

PART 1

Circle the letter corresponding to the appropriate answer.

1. When obtaining information regarding the day history of a child, the nurse should ask:

    A. "How much food does your child normally eat?"

    B. "Does your child socialize well with others?"

    C. "Describe your child's normal sleep patterns."

    D. "What types of stools does your child normally have?"

2. An important nursing consideration when performing a physical assessment on a newborn is to:

    A. prevent squirming.

    B. maintain body temperature.

    C. examine the ears and throat before the eyes and nose.

    D. avoid restraints.

3. When performing an assessment of the throat, depressing the tongue of a child who has acute epiglottiditis is contraindicated because this

    A. may precipitate upper airway obstruction.

    B. overstimulates the cough and gag reflex.

    C. may be a source of bacterial infections.

    D. may rupture the epiglottis.

4. The most effective way to assess a toddler's gait is to

    A. observe play activity.

    B. perform a specific motor test.

    C. ask the child to walk with the parent.

    D. ask the child to hop on one foot.

5. To assess hearing in a 1-month-old infant the nurse should

    A. play a musical toy 4 feet from the infant's ear and observe for eye movement.

    B. repeat the infant's name in a soft tone and observe facial expressions.

    C. perform the Rinne test and observe for head turning.

    D. make a loud noise and observe for the startle reflex.

6. An important reason for assessing the area under the tongue of an adolescent is to

    A. detect early signs of oral cancer.

    B. observe for geographic tongue.

    C. measure the length of the frenulum.

    D. test for Cooper's palsy.

7. An indication of bowel obstruction in the toddler is

    A. increased peristalsis with absence of stools for 2 or more days.

    B. abdominal distention with absence of peristalsis.

    C. severe abdominal pain with a loud bruit on auscultation.

    D. presence of an abdominal hernia with dry, foul-smelling stools.

8. Which of the following statements is correct regarding the assessment findings of the female genitalia?

    A. Hair growth on the mon pubis is a normal finding in children between the ages of 8 and 12.

    B. A vaginal discharge in a young child may be a sign of sexual molestation.

    C. An enlarged clitoris in an adolescent girl is a sign of sexual activity.

    D. Vaginal warts are common findings in most children under the age of 13.

9. What would be an appropriate nursing assessment for a child who complains of a sore throat and dizziness?

    A. Otoscopic and throat exam

    B. Otoscopic and ophthalmic exam

    C. Complete neurologic exam

    D. Respiratory system assessment

10. When performing an assessment for the presence of an inguinal hernia, which of the following should be considered a positive test result?

    A. Palpable femoral lymph nodes

    B. Extreme pain and discomfort in the rectal and perineal area

    C. Bulging of the intestine while coughing

    D. Pelvic pain on palpation

11. To assess the school-age child for scoliosis the nurse should

    A. ask the child to stand straight with feet together.

    B. measure the leg lengths and pelvic girth.

    C. have the child bend over.

    D. ask the child to walk and observe posture.

12. Which of the following statements made by Tina's mother indicates a visual problem?

    A. "Tina is always blinking and squinting."

    B. "Tina does not seem to be interested in her toys."

    C. "Tina tends to bump into things."

    D. "Tina rubs her eyes a lot."

13. To conduct the Denver Articulation Screening Examination (DASE), the nurse would ask Tina to

    A. repeat some familiar words or phrases.

    B. read a favorite short story.

    C. recite a poem with age-appropriate words.

    D. read a phrase and interpret it.

PART 2: CASE STUDY

Jennifer, age 14, is visiting the primary care center for a routine "return to school" physical. She will be examined by the physician to determine her diagnosis and the immediate care necessary.

1. What is an important consideration related to the examination and privacy that the nurse should be aware of regarding Jennifer?

2. On examination, how would the nurse divide the abdomen for inspection?

3. What would be the appearance of the abdomen if the contour and structure are normal?

4. Describe the sounds to be heard on auscultation.

■ Section Four: Inquiry and Exploration

PART 1: CRITICAL INQUIRY EXERCISES

1. Pair off with another nursing student and practice performing an initial assessment using the eight categories for data gathering.

2. There is a significant change in the growth and development of the child moving from a toddler to a preschooler stage of development. Contrast the physical differences that you may find between the two groups of children.

PART 2: CRITICAL EXPLORATION EXERCISES

1. Visit a well-child clinic or pediatrician's office and observe the performance of health assessments on children in various age groups. Focus on communication styles and techniques used by the parent, child, and health care provider.

2. Select a parent group, and explain to them why the Denver Developmental Screening Tool is used and how it is scored and interpreted.

Communication and Teaching With Children and Families

CHAPTER OVERVIEW

Chapter 34 discusses communication and health teaching techniques as related to children, beginning with an overview of nursing process specific to communication with children. Types of learning, the influence of age on learning, and techniques for developing and implementing a teaching plan are included. Health teaching for a surgical experience is used as an example.

LEARNING OBJECTIVES

After mastering the contents of this chapter, you should be able to:

1. Describe the principles of effective communication and teaching and learning as they relate to health teaching with children.

2. Assess children for their ability to communicate and readiness to learn.

3. State nursing diagnoses related to communication and health teaching with children.

4. Identify expected outcomes for a specific child based on the child's age, developmental maturity, emotional needs, and communication or learning style.

5. Plan nursing care based on the use of communication and health teaching priorities.

6. Implement health teaching (e.g., devising a puppet show) using principles of effective communication and teaching-learning.

7. Evaluate outcome criteria to be certain that outcomes established for care have been achieved.

8. Identify National Health Goals related to communicating with and teaching children that nurses could be instrumental in helping the nation achieve.

9. Identify areas of care related to effective communication or health teaching of children that could benefit from additional nursing research or application of evidence-based nursing practice.

10. Use critical thinking to analyze ways that therapeutic communication and health teaching can be further incorporated into the nursing care of children and families.

11. Integrate knowledge of effective communication and teaching-learning with the nursing process to achieve quality maternal and child health nursing care.

KEY TERMS

affective learning
behavior modification
clarifying
cognitive learning
communication
demonstration
empathy
feedback
focusing
health fairs

nontherapeutic communication
paraphrasing
perception checking
positive reinforcement
psychomotor learning
redemonstration
reflecting
teaching plan
therapeutic communication

■ Section One:
Identification of Key Terms and Concepts

PART 1

Match the terms in Part A with a definition or related statement from Part B. Place the letter corresponding to the answer in the space provided. (Letters may be used only once; some letters may not be used.)

PART A

1. _____ Nontherapeutic communication

2. _____ Therapeutic communication

3. _____ Feedback

4. _____ Reflecting

5. _____ Clarifying

6. _____ Perception checking

7. _____ Focusing

PART B

A. Helping someone center on a subject that you suspect is causing anxiety because he or she comments about it indirectly or completely avoids it

B. Interaction that is planned, has structure, and is helpful and constructive

C. Repeating statements someone has made so that you both can be certain you understood

D. Restating the last word or phrase someone has said when there is a pause in the communication

E. Documenting a feeling or emotion that someone has expressed to you

F. Restating what someone has said not only to indicate that you have heard correctly but to help explain what the person is trying to say

G. Interaction that lacks structure, planning, and deliberate purpose

H. A response acknowledging a message has been received and understood

PART 2

Match the terms in Part A with a definition or related statement from Part B. Place the letter corresponding to the answer in the space provided. (Letters may be used only once; some letters may not be used.)

PART A

1. _____ Behavior modification

2. _____ Cognitive learning

3. _____ Informal teaching

4. _____ Learning

5. _____ Lifestyle

6. _____ Psychomotor learning

7. _____ Puppetry

8. _____ Resource people

9. _____ Role modeling

10. _____ Teaching

PART B

A. A two-step process involving the acquisition of knowledge resulting in a measurable change in behavior

B. Requires a change in an individual's ability to perform a skill

C. Involves a change in the individual's level of understanding or knowledge

D. Specific persons in an agency who specialize in teaching particular information or skills

E. A system aimed at erasing some form of activity that interferes with health functioning

F. Presenting information so as to increase someone's knowledge or insight

G. The common pattern of a child's life

H. A helpful method for teaching preschool children about the hospital and health care staff

I. Occurs when a nurse spontaneously answers a child's or parent's question about a care measure

J. Demonstrating a certain attitude that you want a child to learn

K. Involves a change in a person's attitude

■ Section Two: Short Answer and Completion Exercises

PART 1

Complete the following fill-in-the-blank exercises.

1. _____ _____ is a method that examines statements, thoughts, and responses to determine effectiveness with therapeutic communication.

2. Learning occurs best with _____ reinforcement.

3. Teaching in the home gives the nurse an opportunity to assess the child's

    _____ , interactions with _____ _____ , and overall

    _____ _____ .

4. Provide the term for the type of learning described. _____ depends on

    muscle and neurologic coordination. _____ requires adequate

    development, intelligence, and attention span. _____ is gained best

    through role modeling, role playing, or shared-experience discussion.

5. ____ _____ is exact imitation of a demonstrated procedure.

6. Learning goals should reflect the _____ of learning desired and should

    establish _____ and _____ guidelines.

7. Teaching strategies are most effective when they are _____ .

8. The use of flash cards or board games may assist a child in _____

    certain information.

9. Since children often absorb one piece of information at a time, preparation for

    surgery should be taught in _____ .

10. Children learn best those things that hold a particular _____ for them.

11. When teaching a psychomotor skill, always assess the child's _____

    _____ to perform the procedure.

PART 2

Complete the following short answer exercises.

1. Discuss three benefits of group teaching.

2. Discuss the three aspects of the first step in developing a teaching plan.

3. Discuss the benefit of using visual aids when teaching children.

4. Explain the concept of learning ability plateaus.

5. Discuss nursing measures that will help the nation achieve health goals related to preventive health care.

■ Section Three:
Critical Thinking for Application of Essential Concepts

PART 1

Circle the letter corresponding to the appropriate answer.

1. Which of the following indicates appropriate use of teaching-learning principles?
   A. Explaining to a school-age child that the kidney transplant is being done because it will be good for him.
   B. Providing a booklet that encourages a preschool child to eat extra meat because it will help to repair his incision.
   C. Having an infant's mother teach the desired procedure using a game.
   D. Using a firm tone to tell a toddler not to touch her bandage.

2. A child may have the greatest difficulty learning which of the following?
   A. Dietary adjustments
   B. Insulin administration
   C. Colostomy irrigation
   D. Range of motion exercises

3. Which of the following is true about children relative to learning?
   A. One child's learning style may differ from another's.
   B. Admitting your discomfort with teaching a subject will negatively affect learning.
   C. Chronologic age is more indicative of learning capability than mental age.
   D. The older the child, the shorter the attention span.

4. Sally has to teach a group of preschoolers to dial 911. The most effective strategy for this teaching would be

   A. pamphlets.

   B. lecture.

   C. discussion.

   D. demonstration.

5. Which of the following should be included in the teaching-learning process with a young child?

   A. Centering information on the child only, since parents cannot change the child's behavior.

   B. Evaluating if the child is performing the desired behavior when indicated.

   C. Letting the child decide the depth of information to be taught.

   D. Teaching the child special ways to prepare the food on a restricted diet.

PART 2

Determine if the following nursing interventions are appropriate or inappropriate. Indicate your answer by placing an "A" or an "I" in the space provided.

1. _____ Provide a long, clear explanation about procedures to preschool clients to facilitate understanding.

2. _____ Have parents present each time health teaching is performed with adolescents.

3. _____ Offer an immediate, concrete reward to school-age children to encourage learning.

4. _____ Assess the child's family patterns before planning the timing for exercise or medication activities after discharge.

5. _____ Do not use puppets for teaching children.

6. _____ Teach multiple ways of performing a skill the first time you teach the skill.

7. _____ Correct a wrong action by first acknowledging a positive aspect of what the child did or how the child performed the action.

PART 3: CASE STUDY

Six-year-old Raoul Mendelez has been newly diagnosed with diabetes. He understands both English and Spanish, although his parents communicate with him and each other almost exclusively in Spanish.

1. As the nurse caring for Raoul, what communication and teaching techniques will you use to maximize his and his parents' comprehension of the disease and the lifestyle changes it will necessitate?

2. During your first teaching session, you notice the parents are constantly interrupting and questioning Raoul, and they appear anxious. You realize you must modify your teaching plan to improve effectiveness. What adjustments would you make?

3. How might your teaching plan change if Raoul were 16 years old?

4. What effects might Raoul's Hispanic culture have on your communication and teaching plan?

▪ Section Four: Inquiry and Exploration

PART 1: CRITICAL INQUIRY EXERCISES

1. Prepare and execute a teaching plan for an adolescent and a school-age child on some aspect of health maintenance or health promotion. Evaluate the effectiveness of your communication and teaching and note the differences in approach and content needed for each group.

2. Prepare a teaching plan for a toddler related to nutrition. Use a creative approach and evaluate its effectiveness in helping the child learn the content presented.

PART 2: CRITICAL EXPLORATION EXERCISES

Examine the discharge teaching forms or documentation at a local health care facility. Evaluate the clarity of instructions for children of various age groups.

UNIT VII

The Nursing Role in Supporting the Health of Ill Children and Their Families

Nursing Care of the Ill Child and Family

CHAPTER OVERVIEW

Chapter 35 provides an overview of the experience of hospitalization and its effect on children from infancy through adolescence and their families. The meaning of the hospital experience to children is discussed. The role of play therapy in the preparation and care of the hospitalized child is reviewed. The use of the nursing process to plan and provide care for the hospitalized child and the family is reviewed.

LEARNING OBJECTIVES

After mastering the contents of this chapter, you should be able to:

1. Describe the meaning of illness and home care, ambulatory, and in-hospital experiences to children.

2. Assess the impact of an illness, especially one requiring a hospital stay, on a child.

3. Formulate nursing diagnoses related to the stress of illness in children.

4. Establish appropriate outcomes for the ill child.

5. Plan nursing care to reduce the stress of illness, such as helping parents plan for hospitalization or home care.

6. Implement measures such as orientation, education, and therapeutic play to reduce the stress of illness.

7. Evaluate outcomes for achievement and effectiveness of care for the ill child.

8. Identify National Health Goals related to hospitalization or health care that nurses can be instrumental in helping the nation achieve.

9. Identify areas related to illness in children that could benefit from additional nursing research or application of evidence-based practice.

10. Use critical thinking to analyze ways in which illness can be made more family-centered and less traumatic for children.

11. Integrate knowledge about the child's response to illness with the nursing process to achieve quality maternal and child health nursing care.

KEY TERMS

case management nursing	play therapy
calorie counting	primary nursing
direct care	rapid-eye movement (REM) sleep
home care	skilled home care
hospice care	sensory overload
indirect care	sleep deprivation
non-rapid-eye movement (NREM) sleep	therapeutic play

■ Section One: Identification of Key Terms and Concepts

PART 1

Match the terms in Part A with a definition or related statement from Part B. (Use each letter only once; some letters may not be used.)

PART A

1. __E__ Ambulatory setting ✓
2. __H__ Cooperative play ✓
3. __I__ Creative play ✓
4. __D__ Dramatic play ✓
5. __G__ Parallel play ✓
6. __A__ Play ↗ ✗ C
7. __C__ Play therapy ↗ ✗ A
8. __B__ Therapeutic play ✓

(handwritten, circled: 6/8)

PART B

A. A psychoanalytic technique used by psychiatrists to help children understand their feelings, thoughts, and motives

B. A play technique that is divided into three types: energy release, dramatic play, and creative play

C. The "work" of children; a means by which children develop increasing cognitive, psychomotor, and social capabilities

D. Acting out an anxiety situation; most effective with preschoolers

E. Should be stocked with toys that can be played with quickly and by single children

F. Type of play in which children watch play intently but are not actively engaged in it

G. Two children playing side by side but seldom attempting to interact with each other

H. Children playing within an organized structure or competing for a desired goal or outcome

I. The child's drawing a picture or making a list to express emotions or knowledge level

PART 2

Indicate if the following statements are true or false by placing a "T" or "F" in the space provided.

1. __T__ Children are not just small adults. ✓

2. __F__ Children should be told that the doctor will be "taking their tonsils out." ✓

3. __F__ New foods should be introduced to the hospitalized infant to promote growth and development. ✓

4. __F__ School-age children cannot describe symptoms with accuracy.

5. __T__ Children can be depended on to monitor their own care and speak up about incorrect procedures and medications.

6. __T__ Children need more nutrients than adults, and thus may require hospitalization for vomiting or diarrhea when adults would not.

7. __T__ Children tend to respond to disease locally rather than systemically.

8. __F__ Assess patient needs relative to cultural differences by using textbook descriptions of the needs of persons of that culture.

9. __F__ Separation is most damaging to a child between ages 2 months and 3 months.

10. __F__ Children older than age 7 should be told of a pending hospitalization as soon as the parents are aware of it.

■ Section Two: Short Answer and Completion Exercises

PART 1

Complete the following short answer and fill-in-the-blank exercises.

1. __Play__ is one of the most powerful tools available to the nurse in working toward the objective of a successful experience for the hospitalized child.

2. The way children deal with hospitalization is based on the following factors: __perception__ of the event, __support__ __people__ available, and effectiveness of past __coping exper__.

3. List five hazards common to all hospitalization regardless of the reason or length of stay.

fear of injury   *unknown*

separation   *control*

anxiety, uncertain

limits

4. The response of children to illness depends on their *cog. level.*, past *exper.*, and level of *awareness/knowledge*

5. Determine the child's symptoms as much by *observation* as by the child's report.

6. Nurses can help the nation meet health care goals related to mental health of children by helping with assessment of children's *stress* level and reducing the *stress* of the hospitalization.

7. Parents of infants who will be hospitalized should bring the child's *fave toy* with the child to the hospital.

8. The three chief fears of the hospitalized toddler or preschooler are fear of the *mutilation*, *unknown*, and *abandonment*.

9. The school-age child and adolescent should have *clear factual* explanations of what will happen in the hospital.

10. Explanations of procedures to young children are not always successful in relieving stress because

_____.

PART 2

Determine the appropriate age range for the following childhood play activities. Indicate the answer in the space provided.

1. *babies / Infant* _____ Need toys in their cribs such as mobiles

2. *adolescent* _____ Would enjoy watching a soap opera and then discussing the people and their problems

3. *toddler* _____ Need put-in and take-out toys, such as blocks that can be stacked

4. *pre-school* _____ Need quiet toys such as crayons, markers, or books

school-age older child

■ Section Three:
Critical Thinking for Application of Essential Concepts

PART 1

Circle the letter corresponding to the appropriate answer.

1. A 6-year-old is to be admitted to the hospital for an elective surgery. The nurse should advise the parents to tell the child about the surgery how many days before admission to prevent unnecessary worry?

    A. 1

    B. 2

    C. 4

    D. 6

2. The nurse might initiate which of the following interventions when caring for a hospitalized child with a disability or chronic illness?

    A. Avoid using information from previous hospitalizations when planning to prepare the child for the current hospitalization

    B. Help the child avoid contact with peers while hospitalized to decrease self-consciousness and the sense of being different

    C. Limit visiting hours to prevent fatigue of the child

    D. Suggest the child write letters to friends or call family members

3. Alice, age 2 years, is in the intensive care unit with multiple tubes and bandages. Her parents are present frequently but appear reluctant to handle Alice's tubes and bandages, although they asked to feed her at meals. The nurse should do which of the following?

    A. Inform the parents that it is important that they learn to change Alice's dressings and perform this procedure often.

    B. Encourage the parents to irrigate Alice's tubing to make them feel more involved in her plan of care.

    C. Allow the parents to feed Alice and do other care measures as they express interest and comfort.

    D. Limit the parents from performing any care for Alice so they will understand that nurses are capable of fully caring for her.

4. When preparing a child for procedures or surgery, the nurse might do which of the following?

    A. Instruct the child to place the thermometer into his or her arms and hold it there.

    B. Prepare the child for surgery by providing the child with a doll and a small scalpel.

    C. Provide a doll and syringe, alcohol wipes, and a tourniquet to prepare the child for a blood-drawing procedure

    D. To help a child cope with a dressing change, allow the child to hand the sterile gauze to the nurse during the procedure.

5. Which of the following would be an appropriate method for influencing a child to assist with a care measure?

   A. Encourage fluid intake by explaining to the child that fluid will keep him from drying up.

   B. Have the child lift hand weights every 2 hours to strengthen muscles.

   C. Originate board games and crossword puzzles to help the child learn about health teaching.

   D. Place an incentive spirometry machine in front of the child and instruct him or her in deep breathing.

PART 2

Determine if the following nursing interventions are appropriate or inappropriate. Indicate your answer by placing an "A" or an "I" in the space provided.

1. __A__ Say grace before administering a tube feeding if the child commonly says grace before meals.

2. __I__ Stand close to the child, at full adult height, during admission to establish a rapport with the child.

3. __I__ Call the child "sugar" or "sweetie" when addressing him/her to create a warm environment and close relationship.

4. __A__ Determine the child's routines and attempt to adapt the hospital routine as much as possible.

5. __A__ Let the child wear his or her own clothes if possible rather than change to a hospital gown.

6. __A__ Limit the number of readmissions and length of stay by teaching parents how to safely monitor their child after a procedure.

7. __A__ Encourage younger siblings to visit, as well as siblings over the age of 12 or 14 years.

8. __I__ Use a team nursing approach to provide the child with a variety of caregivers.

9. __I__ Perform procedures such as blood drawing at the bedside to establish this area as the child's care area.

10. __A__ Allow the child to make as many decisions during a procedure as possible to facilitate a sense of control.

PART 3: CASE STUDY

Devon, a 3-year-old who had emergency surgery while on vacation, has been separated from her single mother, who had to return home because of her job, and 14-year-old sister. Devon has been without her family for 4 days.

1. What behaviors would you expect Devon to display to nursing staff over the next days?

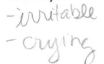

   –irritable

   –crying

2. What effect might Devon's hospitalization and absence have on her mother and older sister?

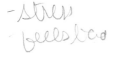

3. What interventions might you plan for Devon and her family?

▪ Section Four: Inquiry and Exploration

PART 1: CRITICAL INQUIRY EXERCISES

1. What measures would you take to prepare a 4-month-old infant and family members for open heart surgery? How would this preparation differ if the surgery were minor?

2. Design a teaching plan for parents whose 2-year-old child will be admitted to the hospital for surgery.

PART 2: CRITICAL EXPLORATION EXERCISES

1. While on a pediatric clinical unit, assess children in varying age groups. Determine if separation anxiety is present, and note the age levels of the children experiencing the highest levels of anxiety.

2. Interview the parent of a hospitalized child. Determine the type of preparation the parent used before bringing the child to the hospital.

Nursing Care of the Child Undergoing Diagnostic Techniques and Other Therapeutic Modalities

CHAPTER OVERVIEW

Chapter 36 provides an overview of the nursing care required for the ill child and family during diagnostic and therapeutic procedures. Adaptations required for children when undergoing diagnostic procedures and various therapeutic techniques are discussed. The use of the nursing process to plan and provide care for the hospitalized child and the family is explored.

LEARNING OBJECTIVES

After mastering the contents of this chapter, you should be able to:

1. Describe common nursing interventions used in the health care of children to aid diagnosis and therapy.

2. Assess children as to developmental stage and knowledge level before beginning diagnostic or therapeutic procedures or other nursing interventions.

3. Formulate nursing diagnoses related to common diagnostic or therapeutic procedures used with children.

4. Identify outcomes for the child undergoing a diagnostic or therapeutic procedure.

5. Plan nursing interventions to aid in diagnosis or therapy for children.

6. Implement nursing interventions relevant to diagnostic or therapeutic procedures.

7. Evaluate outcomes related to diagnostic and therapeutic procedures for achievement.

8. Identify National Health Goals related to diagnostic and therapeutic procedures for children that nurses could be instrumental in helping the nation achieve.

9. Identify areas related to nursing procedures with children that could benefit from additional nursing research or application of evidence-based practice.

10. Use critical thinking to analyze ways that diagnostic and therapeutic procedures can be modified to meet the needs of children.

11. Integrate knowledge of common diagnostic and therapeutic procedures with nursing process to achieve quality maternal and child health nursing.

KEY TERMS

aspiration studies	gavage feedings
barium contrast studies	magnetic resonance imaging (MRI)
bronchoscopy	positron emission tomography (PET)
clean-catch urine specimen	radiopharmaceutical
colonoscopy	single photon emission computerized
computed tomography (CT)	tomography (SPECT)
electrical impulse studies	total parenteral nutrition (TPN)
endoscopy	ultrasound

■ Section One:
Identification of Key Terms and Concepts

Match the terms in Part A with a definition or related statement from Part B. Place the letter corresponding to the answer in the space provided.

PART A

1. _____ Barium contrast studies

2. _____ Gavage feedings

3. _____ Total parenteral nutrition (TPN)

4. _____ Bronchoscopy

5. _____ Radiopharmaceutical

PART B

A. Infusion of a concentrated hypertonic solution into a central or peripheral intravenous site

B. Radioactive-combined substances that when given orally or by injection flow to designated body organs for a diagnostic picture

C. Direct visualization of the larynx, trachea, and bronchi through a fiberoptic tube

D. Use of radiopaque dye to outline the gastrointestinal tract

E. Supplying adequate nutrition through a nasogastric tube

■ Section Two:
Short Answer and Completion Exercises

PART 1

Complete the following fill-in-the-blank exercises.

1. A _____-_____ specimen involves collecting urine after usual voiding after the external meatus has been cleaned.

2. Two problems when using an ostomy appliance with an infant are

   _____ and _____ _____.

3. Restraints should be checked every _____ minutes to ensure that circulation is intact.

4. When securing a dressing on infants and young children, use _____ tape.

PART 2

Complete the following short answer exercises.

1. Discuss the psychological and physical preparation needed for a child undergoing surgery.

2. List four common types of restraints used with children.

_____   _____

_____   _____

3. Describe two ways in which nurses can help the nation achieve goals related to reducing the length of hospital stay for children.

■ Section Three:
Critical Thinking for Application of Essential Concepts

PART 1

Circle the letter corresponding to the appropriate answer.

1. When a procedure is being performed that requires a consent form, which of the following is true?

   A. A consent form can be omitted if the procedure involves only a minimal risk.

   B. The nurse must explain the procedure and obtain signed consent if the physician does not.

   C. Emancipated minors must have parental permission to sign a consent form.

   D. In single-parent families, the custodial parent must sign the consent form.

2. The nurse's role in assisting with diagnostic procedures includes which of the following?

   A. Helping the child to forget the experience of the procedure as quickly as possible

   B. Using complex medical terms to explain procedures to children and parents to demonstrate knowledge and competence

    C. Explaining the preparation and actual procedure before beginning either

    D. Sending mature children to different test departments without supervision to increase independence

3. Which of the following is appropriate when modifying procedures for children?

    A. Parents should be asked to restrain infants when indicated.

    B. Toddlers should be given procedures quickly and without warning to decrease resistance.

    C. Adolescents should be expected to tolerate procedures maturely and without fear.

    D. School-age children should be given thorough explanations for procedures.

4. When performing contrast dye studies with children, the nurse should

    A. tell the child the flavored barium will taste like a milkshake to increase cooperation.

    B. isolate the child after the test until the radioactivity resolves.

    C. explain to the child that a warm feeling may be experienced with IV dye.

    D. restrict all activity for the duration of the procedure to prevent distracting the child.

5. When teaching parents about temperature reduction in children, the nurse should include which of the following interventions?

    A. Administer acetylsalicylic acid every 4 hours until the child's temperature is less than 101°F.

    B. Dress the child in warm flannel night clothes to prevent chilling.

    C. Give a full dose of ibuprofen (Motrin) to reduce temperature.

    D. Place an ice cloth on the child's forehead and refresh it every hour.

6. After an endoscopy study, which of the following interventions would be most important?

    A. Pushing oral fluids immediately to promote elimination of dye

    B. Monitoring airway and respiratory function for the first 4 hours

    C. Applying a warm compress to the neck to reduce spasm

    D. Administering atropine to reduce pulmonary secretions

PART 2

Determine if the following nursing interventions are appropriate or inappropriate. Indicate your answer by placing an "A" or an "I" in the space provided.

1. _____ Allowing the child to look at the incision during a dressing change

2. _____ Taking a radial pulse for children under 1 year of age

3. _____ Cuddling and calming an infant before assessing respiratory rate

4. _____ Taking an axillary or tympanic temperature in children from infancy to age 4

5. _____ Assessing blood pressure in routine assessment of children over 3 years of age

6. _____ Recognizing that in children it is normal to have a thigh blood pressure lower than the blood pressure in the arms

7. _____ Drawing a child's blood at the bedside to decrease the trauma of the experience

8. _____ Attaching a collection bag to a child who has not been toilet trained to collect a urine specimen

9. _____ Pushing children to drink several glasses of fluid before voiding for a urine specimen

10. _____ Sponging children with cold water to lower the temperature

11. _____ Explaining to a school-age child that an ultrasound will be painful but is a necessary diagnostic procedure

12. _____ Telling a preschool child a shot will hurt for only a short time

13. _____ Praising a child for cooperation even if none was visibly obvious

14. _____ Instructing adolescents on the cleaning procedure for clean-catch specimens

PART 3: CASE STUDY

Iesha Jackson, age 2, is admitted to your care after stabilization of a sickle cell crisis. She is screaming for her mother and trying to get out of bed. Her mother, age 18, is in the waiting room making a call. She says Iesha's father is the custodial parent and this crisis happened on "her weekend" with Iesha. She doesn't want to call Iesha's father for fear he will blame her.

1. Iesha will require several invasive procedures during her stay. What teaching responsibilities do you have in this situation?

2. How will the fact that Iesha's parents are separated affect your discharge teaching plan?

■ Section Four: Inquiry and Exploration

PART 1: CRITICAL INQUIRY EXERCISES

1. Review five skills listed in a fundamentals text that were not discussed in this chapter, and note ways in which those skills might need to be adjusted for an infant or child.

2. Plan a schedule for a 4-year-old child who must have blood drawn for lab work, an abdominal x-ray, a CT scan, and an endoscopy during her 2-day hospital stay.

PART 2: CRITICAL EXPLORATION EXERCISES

Tour a pediatric unit and observe the procedures being performed. Compare the techniques used with those noted on an adult floor, and note any variations.

Nursing Care of the Child Undergoing Medication Administration and Intravenous Therapy

CHAPTER OVERVIEW

Chapter 37 provides an overview of the nursing care required for the ill child and family regarding medication administration and intravenous therapy. Adaptations required for children during the preparation and administration of medications and when planning and implementing intravenous therapy are discussed. The use of the nursing process to plan and provide care for the child and the family involved in medication administration and intravenous therapy is explored.

LEARNING OBJECTIVES

After mastering the contents of this chapter, you should be able to:

1. Describe common methods of medication administration used in the health care of children.

2. Assess the developmental stage and knowledge level of children and adolescents before beginning medication administration.

3. Formulate nursing diagnoses related to medication administration with children.

4. Identify outcomes for children receiving medication.

5. Plan nursing interventions to aid in making medicine administration maximally effective.

6. Implement nursing interventions concerned with medication administration and children.

7. Evaluate outcomes related to medication administration with children.

8. Identify National Health Goals related to medication administration that nurses could be instrumental in helping the nation achieve.

9. Identify areas related to medication administration with children that could benefit from additional nursing research or application of evidence-based practice.

10. Use critical thinking to analyze ways that medication administration can be modified to meet the needs of children of all ages.

11. Integrate knowledge of medication administration with nursing process to achieve quality maternal and child health nursing.

KEY TERMS

absorption	intermittent infusion devices
distribution	metabolism
excretion	pharmacokinetics
Intracath	vascular access port

■ Section One:
Identification of Key Terms and Concepts

Match the terms in Part A with a definition or related statement from Part B. Place the letter corresponding to the answer in the space provided.

PART A

1. _____ Absorption

2. _____ Distribution

3. _____ Intracath

4. _____ Metabolism

5. _____ Pharmacokinetics

PART B

A. a slim, pliable catheter threaded into a vein; used for long periods of intravenous therapy

B. the way a drug is absorbed, distributed throughout the body, metabolized, inactivated, and excreted

C. conversion of the drug into an active form or an inactive form

D. movement of the drug through the bloodstream to a specific site of action

E. transfer of the drug from its point of entry into the bloodstream

■ Section Two:
Short Answer and Completion Exercises

PART 1

Complete the following fill-in-the-blank exercises.

1. Four routes by which medications are given to children are _____ ,

   _____ , _____ , or _____ .

2. Before administering any medication to a child, confirm that the dose ordered

   is correct for the child's _____ or _____ _____ .

3. When administering nose drops, place the child on his or her _____ .

4. To administer ear drops to a child under 2 years, straighten the ear canal by

   pulling the pinna _____ and _____ .

5. The mandatory site for intramuscular injections in infants is the _____ _____.

6. _____ therapy is the quickest and most effective means of administering fluid or medicine to the ill infant or child.

7. A _____ _____ can be used to draw frequent venous blood samples.

8. The _____ of body systems in infants and children plays a major role in drug action.

PART 2

Complete the following short answer exercises.

1. Discuss how age may alter drug absorption, distribution, inactivation, and excretion.

2. Explain circumstances under which restraints may be used with infants and children during intravenous therapy.

3. List three fluid infusion safety measures to be used with children.

   _____   _____

   _____

4. The six rights of medication administration are Right: _____ , _____ , _____ , _____ , _____ , and _____.

■ Section Three:
Critical Thinking for Application of Essential Concepts

PART 1

Circle the letter corresponding to the appropriate answer.

1. Sites frequently used for intravenous insertion in young children or infants include which of the following?
   A. Antecubital and veins on the extensor surface of the wrist
   B. Jugular and veins on the ventral surface of the hand

C. Veins located in the leg or on the surface of the foot

D. Radial or ulnar surface veins or the subclavian vein

2. The nurse preparing to initiate intravenous therapy with a 1-year-old infant would obtain which of the following size catheters?

A. 16-gauge

B. 18-gauge

C. 20-gauge

D. 22-gauge

3. A child weighing 20 kg is to begin fluid therapy. Using Table 37-1 and based on caloric expenditure, the child should receive how many milliliters of maintenance solution containing 5% dextrose, 25 mEq sodium, and 20 mEq of potassium per liter?

A. 1,500

B. 1,725

C. 2,000

D. 2,300

4. The nurse can be instrumental in helping the nation achieve national health goals related to children and drugs or medication administration by

A. stressing the importance of using medications to treat every discomfort.

B. educating parents regarding the importance of steroid use to treat acne in adolescents.

C. teaching stress management techniques to children and parents for use to address anxiety.

D. instructing parents to keep medication at the bedside for ease of access.

5. A 3-year-old child may receive a medication dosage consistent with the dosage usually given to a 1-year-old if the 3-year-old child:

A. was developmentally delayed.

B. was tall for his/her age.

C. had the surface area of a 1-year-old.

D. weighed more than a 1-year-old.

6. When assessing a child before medication administration, it is important to determine which of the following?

A. The child's dosage preference

B. Past medication-taking experiences

C. Parental developmental status

D. Whether the medication is having the desired effect

PART 2

Determine if the following nursing interventions are appropriate or inappropriate.
Indicate your answer by placing an "A" or an "I" in the space provided.

1. _____ Instructing parents to store drugs in locked, elevated cabinets

2. _____ Asking a child, "Will you drink this for me?" to help the child feel respected

3. _____ Telling the child it is time to take the medicine and asking the child's preference of water or milk to take the medicine with

4. _____ Mixing bitter medicine with a large glass of juice to dilute the taste

5. _____ Crushing a tablet and mixing it with applesauce for better taste when appropriate

6. _____ Offering a preschooler or older child a choice of location for insertion of an IV when possible

7. _____ Telling a preschool child a shot will hurt for only a short time

8. _____ Providing oral medications to children under 3 years of age in tablet form

9. _____ Avoiding referring to a child's medicine as candy

10. _____ Asking a child his or her name for identification before administering medications

PART 3: CASE STUDY

India Jeilhal is admitted to your care after a playground accident. The 5-year-old is sitting up in bed holding her mother's hand. The doctor has ordered an IV to infuse an antibiotic as well as oral pain medication. India's mother is asking you to give India something for pain.

1. How would you respond to India's mother's request? What teaching responsibilities do you have in this situation?

2. How will you prepare for the initiation of intravenous therapy? What measures will you take to prepare India and her mother for the procedure?

■ Section Four: Inquiry and Exploration

PART 1: CRITICAL INQUIRY EXERCISES

1. Discuss ways in which you might need to alter your approach when administering an intramuscular injection to a 1-month-old, a 1-year-old, a 5-year-old, a 10-year-old, or a 16-year-old child.

2. Plan instructions for the parents of a 4-year-old child who must administer an oral medication that comes in tablet form only.

PART 2: CRITICAL EXPLORATION EXERCISES

Tour a neonatal unit and pediatric unit and observe intravenous therapy in place with children of various ages. Compare the techniques and equipment used with the different age groups.

Pain Management in Children

CHAPTER OVERVIEW

Chapter 38 discusses the management of pain in children. The causes of pain as well as the assessment and measurement of pain are discussed, with emphasis on developmental considerations. Varied pain management strategies are reviewed, including pharmacologic and nonpharmacologic measures. The use of the nursing process to plan and provide appropriate care and teaching to promote appropriate pain management in children is discussed.

LEARNING OBJECTIVES

After mastering the contents of this chapter, you should be able to:

1. Describe the major methods of pain management in children.

2. Use the nursing process to identify physical and psychological aspects of care required for the child who is in pain and to plan and implement that care.

3. Identify National Health Goals related to children with pain that nurses could be instrumental in helping the nation achieve.

4. Use critical thinking to analyze ways that nursing care for a child with pain could be more family-centered.

5. Integrate knowledge of pain in children with the nursing process to achieve quality child health nursing care.

KEY TERMS

acute pain
chronic pain
conscious sedation
distraction
epidural analgesia
gate control theory
imagery

pain
pain threshold
patient-controlled analgesia
referred pain
substitution of meaning
thought stopping
transcutaneous electrical nerve stimulation

■ Section One:
Identification of Key Terms and Concepts

Match the terms in Part A with a definition or related statement from Part B. Place the letter corresponding to the answer in the space provided.

PART A

1. __D__ Distraction

2. __C__ Gate control theory

3. __E__ Patient-controlled analgesia
4. __A__ Thought stopping
5. __B__ Transcutaneous electrical nerve stimulation

PART B

A. a technique whereby children are taught to substitute a positive or relaxing thought for anxious thoughts

B. use of a current to interfere with the transmission of the pain impulse across small nerve fibers

C. explains how pain impulses travel between a site of injury and the brain, where the impulse is actually registered as pain

D. allows the cells of the brain stem that register an impulse as pain to be preoccupied with other stimuli so the pain impulse cannot register

E. allows a child to self-administer IV opiate boluses with a medication pump to control pain

■ Section Two: Short Answer and Completion Exercises

PART 1

Complete the following fill-in-the-blank exercises.

1. The technique that allows the child to be both pain-free and sedated for a procedure and leaves protective reflexes intact is called _conscious sedation_.

2. To reduce the pain of procedures such as venipuncture or lumbar puncture, a _topical anesthetic_ cream may be applied.

3. _oral analgesia_ is an advantageous and cost-effective pain control method that is relatively easy to administer.

4. A numerical or _visual analog_ scale uses a straight line with end points marked 0 for no pain on the left and 10 for worst pain on the right.

5. _Substitution of meaning_ or imagery is a distraction technique that helps a child place another, nonpainful meaning on a painful procedure.

PART 2

Complete the following short answer exercises.

1. Discuss two of three reasons that nurses do not provide adequate pain relief to children.

2. Explain why pain assessment might be difficult with children.

3. Briefly discuss the gate control theory.

▪ Section Three:
Critical Thinking for Application of Essential Concepts

PART 1

Circle the letter corresponding to the appropriate answer.

1. When assessing the pain of an infant, the nurse should consider which of the following?
   A. Infants are preverbal, so cues such as tears or guarding a body part can be helpful.
   B. Infants will be comforted completely only by a parent if the pain is very intense.
   C. An infant can indicate if he or she has pain and exactly where the pain is located.
   D. Since infants think concretely, they may associate words like "sharp" with knives.

2. Which of the following is true about pain assessment for the school-age child and adolescent?
   A. A scale of 1 to 10 should be used for younger children to provide the child with maximum choices.
   B. Some children may require preassessment work to evaluate if they understand incremental measurements.
   C. School-age children use mechanisms for controlling pain that are unique and different from adult mechanisms.
   D. Preadolescents think very concretely, so they can describe pain with little difficulty.

3. Which of the following tools allows the health care provider to rate pain without the need of self-report input by the child and incorporates five behaviors usually seen with pain?

   A. Logs and diaries of pain episodes

   B. Oucher pain rating scale

   C. FLACC pain assessment tool

   D. Poker chip tool

4. Analgesia instilled in the space just outside the spinal canal is called

   A. local anesthesia.

   B. epidural analgesia.

   C. intranasal analgesia.

   D. intravenous analgesia.

PART 2: CASE STUDY

Patricia Walters, age 4, is admitted onto your unit after having her tonsils removed. Her mother is concerned that Patricia might have pain but says she is afraid of injections.

1. Patricia's mother asks if you will need to hold Patricia down because she hates needles but needs something for pain. What are some responses you might give?

2. What are some methods you might use to assess Patricia's pain? Which pain assessment tools would be inappropriate?

■ Section Four: Inquiry and Exploration

PART 1: CRITICAL INQUIRY EXERCISES

1. What key points would you address in a teaching plan for a school-age child and parents when the child is discharged home after a painful day surgery? In addition to pain medication, what other pain relief measures might you include in this teaching plan?

2. What should you do if a school-age child or adolescent who is 1 day post surgery and has had no pain medication since surgery denies pain but shows signs of discomfort?

PART 2: CRITICAL EXPLORATION EXERCISES

Visit a pediatric cancer unit and a postoperative inpatient care unit at a pediatric hospital. Compare the pain control methods used on each unit. Note the route of administration and the types of analgesics used.

The Nursing Role in Restoring and Maintaining the Health of Children and Families With Physiologic Disorders

Nursing Care of the Child Born With a Physical Developmental Disorder

CHAPTER OVERVIEW

Chapter 39 reviews several defects seen among children and examines nursing strategies and implementations used during therapy and corrective and surgical procedures. This chapter also assists students in synthesizing the knowledge needed to formulate appropriate nursing care plans and evaluate the outcome of nursing goals for children with physical developmental disorders. A case study guides the student in assessing and determining proper nursing interventions for a client with a spinal and neurologic defect.

LEARNING OBJECTIVES

After mastering the contents of this chapter, you should be able to:

1. Describe common physical developmental birth disorders.

2. Assess a newborn who is born physically challenged.

3. Develop nursing diagnoses for the child with a physical developmental disorder.

4. Establish outcomes to meet the needs of the child with a physical developmental disorder.

5. Plan nursing care to meet the established outcomes of care for the child born with a physical developmental disorder.

6. Carry out nursing interventions for care of children born with physical developmental disorders, such as preventing infection in the child with spina bifida.

7. Evaluate outcomes to determine achievement and effectiveness of care.

8. Identify National Health Goals related to children born with physical disabilities that nurses could be instrumental in helping the nation achieve.

9. Identify areas related to developmentally challenged infants that could benefit by additional nursing research or application of evidence-based practice.

10. Use critical thinking to analyze the impact of a developmentally challenged child on the family and propose ways to make care more family-centered.

11. Integrate knowledge of congenital physical anomalies with the nursing process to achieve quality maternal and child health nursing care.

KEY TERMS

ankyloglossia	meconium plug
atresia	omphalocele
cleft lip	polydactyly
cleft palate	spina bifida
developmental hip dysplasia	stenosis
fistula	syndactyly
frenulum	transillumination
hydrocephalus	volvulus

■ Section One: Identification of Key Terms and Concepts

Match the terms in Part A with a definition or related statement from Part B. (Use each letter only once; some letters may not be used.)

PART A

1. _____ Ankyloglossia

2. _____ Pierre Robin syndrome

3. _____ Diaphragmatic hernia

4. _____ Torticollis

5. _____ Meconium ileus

6. _____ Hydrocephalus

7. _____ Craniosynostosis

8. _____ Thyroglossal

9. _____ Polydactyly

10. _____ Umbilical hernia

11. _____ Talipes

12. _____ Achondroplasia

13. _____ Microcephaly

14. _____ Atresia

15. _____ Gastroschisis

16. _____ Fistula

17. _____ Frenulum

PART B

A. slow brain growth resulting in mental retardation

B. occurs in newborns who are later diagnosed with cystic fibrosis due to absent enzyme

C. a cyst that arises from an embryogenic fault; anterior portion of the neck fails to close

D. protrusion of abdominal organs into the chest cavity through a defect in the diaphragm

E. restriction of the tongue caused by an abnormally tight frenulum

F. birth defect identified as a trait anomaly-small mandible, cleft palate, and glossoptosis

G. defect in cartilage production resulting in dwarfism

H. protrusion of a portion of the intestine through umbilical ring, muscle, fascia

I. one or more additional fingers

J. ankle-foot deformity

K. occurs when sternocleidomastoid muscle sustains injury during birth; infant holds head tilted to the side

L. premature closure of sutures of the skull

M. congenital deformity of the scapulae; one scapula is turned horizontally

N. opening in the esophagus leading to the trachea

O. membrane attached to lower anterior tip of tongue

P. absence of canalization in the bowel, where complete closure may occur

Q. an excess of cerebrospinal fluid in the ventricles and subarachnoid spaces of the brain

R. herniation of abdominal contents without peritoneal membrane to contain it

■ Section Two:
Short Answer and Completion Exercises

Complete the following fill-in-the-blank exercises.

1. _____ is the absence of the cerebral hemisphere of the brain.

2. _____ _____ deformity is due to an overgrowth of the neural tube in the 16th to 20th week of fetal growth.

3. A _____ _____ is a hard portion of meconium completely obstructing the intestinal lumen.

4. _____ is the audible noise heard when the femoral head dislocates from the acetabular roof.

5. _____ and _____ are the two types of congenital hip dysplasia.

■ Section Three:
Critical Thinking for Application of Essential Concepts

PART 1

Circle the letter corresponding to the appropriate answer.

1. Leonard, age 8 months, is visiting the health clinic for a well-baby check-up. He is diagnosed with congenital hip dysplasia. The physician describes the defect as no communication between the femoral head and the acetabulum. This dysplasia is called

   A. preluxation.

   B. subluxation.

   C. dislocation.

   D. acetabular subluxation.

2. A nurse performing the assessment on an infant with hip dysplasia would find that the affected extremity

   A. appears slightly shorter than the normal one.

   B. is resistant to extension.

   C. will not allow the child to lie supine with feet flexed.

   D. is obviously malformed.

3. Dayle is a 3-month-old admitted to the hospital with a diagnosis of hydro-cephalus. Which of the following are signs of increased intracranial pressure?

   A. Overriding sutures

   B. Poor sucking

   C. Hyper reflex activity

   D. Prominent scalp veins

4. After a shunt to relieve intracranial pressure, which of the following would indicate an infection?

   A. Subnormal temperature

   B. Decreased pulse

   C. Marked irritability

   D. Supple neck

5. Desmond is admitted to the surgical floor of the pediatric hospital several hours after birth for a tracheoesophageal fistula. The nurse may observe atypical characteristics such as

   A. constantly blowing mucus bubbles from the mouth.

   B. absence of stools.

   C. absence of rooting reflex.

   D. inability to swallow.

6. Crying is to be avoided in a child who has had a cleft lip repair because it

   A. sustains a traumatic experience.

   B. places tension on the suture line.

   C. threatens maternal-infant bonding.

   D. predisposes to respiratory difficulties.

7. When caring for an infant with a meningocele, the nurse should
   A. place a pillow under the infant's head.
   B. position the infant supine with the head of bed at 45 degrees.
   C. place plastic on the child's back under the meningocele.
   D. replace the wet compress every 4 hours with a fresh saline compress.

8. After repair of a tracheoesophageal fistula, the nurse would watch the infant carefully at postoperative days 7 to 10 for which of the following symptoms of leaks at anastomosis sites?
   A. Serous drainage
   B. Acute indigestion
   C. Profuse diarrhea
   D. Respiratory distress

PART 2: CASE STUDY

Patrick is approximately 24 hours old. The doctors are implementing tests and procedures to determine if his congenital neural tube defect is a meningocele or a myelomeningocele.

1. How does a meningocele different from a myelomeningocele?

2. What are the physical characteristics that Patrick would exhibit if diagnosed with a myelomeningocele?

3. Preoperatively, Patrick should be placed in what position?

4. The nurse should give special attention to Patrick's elimination status. What procedure might the nurse implement to aid in bladder elimination?

■ Section Four: Inquiry and Exploration

PART 1: CRITICAL INQUIRY EXERCISES

1. Create a teaching plan for parents to perform a neurologic assessment on a child discharged from the hospital in a spica cast.

2. Identify the major components of the assessment when examining an infant for a diaphragmatic hernia. What are the physiologic explanations for the positive findings that you might find on assessment?

PART 2: CRITICAL EXPLORATION EXERCISES

1. Visit the physical therapy department at your clinical facility. Identify the equipment used for motor development by the patients in the hospital and by the patients who visit for outpatient therapy.

2. Visit a community agency that sponsors the annual Special Olympics in your area. Speak with an appropriate staff member to learn some basic psychosocial skills on how to communicate with and motivate the child who has a chronic physical developmental defect.

CHAPTER 40

Nursing Care of the Child With a Respiratory Disorder

CHAPTER OVERVIEW

Respiratory diseases are serious in children because the lumens of respiratory structures are small in children and likely to become obstructed in disease. Nurses need good assessment skills to assess clinical status. This chapter presents the most common disorders of the upper and lower respiratory tract, along with their therapeutic management. Care that incorporates the provision of airway patency by administering aerosols and bronchodilators, postural drainage and position changes, and antibiotics for infection is also addressed.

LEARNING OBJECTIVES

After mastering the contents of this chapter, you should be able to:

1. Describe common respiratory illnesses in children.

2. Assess the child with a respiratory illness.

3. Use the nursing process to formulate and address nursing diagnoses related to respiratory illness in children.

4. Identify National Health Goals related to children with respiratory disorders that nurses could be instrumental in helping the nation achieve.

5. Identify areas related to care of children with respiratory disorders that could benefit from additional nursing research.

6. Use critical thinking to analyze ways that nursing care for a child with a respiratory illness could be more family-centered.

7. Synthesize knowledge of respiratory illness in children with the nursing process to achieve quality maternal and child health nursing care.

KEY TERMS

adventitious sounds
aspiration
atelectasis
bronchial breathing
clubbing
cupping
cyanosis
expiration
hypoxemia
hypoxia
inspiration

paroxysmal coughing
percussion
pneumothorax
postural drainage
rales
retraction
stridor
tachypnea
vesicular breathing
wheezing

■ Section One:
Identification of Key Terms and Concepts

Match the terms in Part A with a definition or related statement from Part B. Place the letter corresponding to the answer in the space provided.

PART A

1. _D_ Hypoxia
2. _C_ Dyspnea
3. _H_ Hypoventilation
4. _A_ Apnea
5. _B_ Hyperventilation
6. _E_ Anoxia
7. _F_ Tachypnea
8. _G_ Hypoxemia
9. _K_ Bronchopulmonary dysplasia
10. _J_ Laryngeal stridor
11. _I_ Rales
12. _L_ Wheezing

Hypox = low O₂ content

Anox = low O₂ tissues

12/12

PART B

A. lack of respiration
B. rapid deep breathing
C. difficulty in respiratory exchange
D. low oxygen content in tissues
E. reduction below adequate levels of oxygen in tissue
F. rapid respiration
G. deficit oxygen content in the blood
H. shallow breathing
I. fine crackling sounds
J. strident sound heard on inspiration
K. a chronic lung condition seen in infants with acute respiratory distress at birth
L. obstruction of lower trachea or bronchioles on expiration; an expiratory sound

■ Section Two:
Short Answer and Completion Exercises

Complete the following fill-in-the-blank and short answer exercises.

1. The respiratory centers are located in the _medulla_ and the _pons_ .

2. The upper respiratory tract functions to _filter_ , _warm_ , and _moisten_ air.

3. The first indicator of airway obstruction in children is _tachypnea_

4. Five common terms used to describe respiratory dysfunctions are _hypoxia_ , _dyspnea_ , _hyper/hypo ventilation_ _tachypnea_ , and _apnea_ .

5. Normal values for each of these blood gas components are P_{O_2} _80-100 mmHg_ , P_{CO_2} _35-45 mmHg_ , O_2 saturation _95-100%_, pH _7.35-7.45_ , and HCO_3 _22-26 mEq/L_

6. The most dangerous periods following a tonsillectomy are the _first 24 hr_ , and the _5th_ to _7th_ day.

7. If a child has no complications following a tonsillectomy, he or she is discharged the same day or the following morning. Three danger signs you would tell the parents to watch for are ↑ _restlessness_ , _swallowing_ , and _clearing throat_ .

8. Children with symptoms of epiglottitis should never be examined with a tongue blade because the gagging might cause _complete_ _obstruction of the glottis_ .

9. Three symptoms of epiglottitis are _sore throat_ , _hoarseness_ , and _high fever_ .

10. Nurses can help the nation achieve health goals focused on respiratory illness in children by teaching children to avoid _smoking_ , by teaching programs to help children with asthma learn ways of _↑_ _activity_ and take steps to reduce the severity of an attack, and by encouraging parents to come for _health maintenance_ visits.

■ Section Three:
Critical Thinking for Application of Essential Concepts

PART 1

Circle the letter corresponding to the appropriate answer.

1. A newborn is showing signs of respiratory distress. How would you assess for choanal atresia? — closure

    A. Make the newborn cry, then gently compress one nostril, then the second.

    B. Compress both nostrils at the same time and open the newborn's mouth.

    C. Hold the newborn's mouth closed, then compress one nostril, then the second.

    D. Have the newborn suck on a bottle as you compress the nostrils.

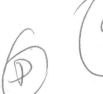
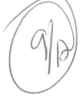

2. Baby Jane was diagnosed with acute nasopharyngitis (common cold). Her mother is going to use a bulb syringe and a vaporizer to clear the congestion. You should teach the mother that

    A. the bulb should be compressed before inserting the syringe into the child's nostril.

    B. the vaporizer should be kept at the bedside so the mist will be close to the child's face.

    C. the vaporizer will not require cleaning since the steam is very hot and sterile.

    D. the bulb syringe should be filled with saline nose drops that should be squeezed into the nostril.

3. Baby John was admitted with streptococcal pharyngitis. When he was discharged, his mother was told to return to the doctor's office in 2 weeks with a urine specimen. The urine would mostly be examined

    A. for fat and lipids to see if the kidneys are working.

    B. for protein to determine if acute glomerulonephritis is developing.

    C. to determine if the child is developing otitis media.

    D. to determine if the child should be kept on a liquid diet or progressed to a soft diet.

4. Nursing care of the child who has had a tonsillectomy should include all of the following except

    A. observing for signs of bleeding.

    B. pushing ice cream hourly to soothe the child's throat.

    C. placing the child on his or her abdomen with a pillow under the chest.

    D. observing for excessive swallowing and throat clearing.

5. If bleeding occurs in a child following a tonsillectomy, the nursing action would be to

    A. elevate the child's head and turn him or her on his or her side.

    B. place the child in a prone position.

    C. place the child in a Trendelenburg position.

    D. elevate the child's feet and turn him or her in a prone position.

6. Which of the following should be given to a child following a tonsillectomy?

    A. Sips of clear liquid or ice chips

    B. Milkshakes or scoops of ice cream

    C. French fries

    D. Popcorn

7. Elisa, a 14-month-old, is admitted to the hospital with laryngotracheobronchitis (croup). On assessment the nurse would expect to find

    A. cyanosis and dyspnea.

    B. productive coughing and a high fever.

    C. pale laryngeal tissue and dyspnea.

    D. barking cough and inspiratory stridor.

8. It is very important that the nurse prevent aspiration following bronchoscopy. Which of the following interventions would be appropriate?

    A. Feed slowly for the first hour.

    B. Keep NPO until the gag reflex has returned.

    C. Keep NPO and provide postural drainage for the first postoperative day.

    D. Keep head elevated at 45 degrees for the first postoperative day.

9. The plan of care for a child with bronchitis should include

    A. bed rest and minimal oral fluid intake.

    B. keeping room air cool and dry.

    C. shallow inspiration to decrease chest pain.

    D. expectorants and coughing to clear secretions.

10. A 5-month-old child is admitted to your unit with bronchiolitis, temperature 102°F, apical pulse 154, respirations 68, and irritability. Oxygen therapy is ordered to

    A. liquefy secretions.

    B. promote rest.

    C. relieve hypoxia and cyanosis.

    D. decrease coughing.

11. All of the following statements are true about cystic fibrosis except:

    A. It is inherited as an autosomal recessive trait.

    B. It occurs in about 1 in 2,000 births, mostly among whites.

    C. Symptoms include patchy consolidations and tumors throughout the lungs.

    D. It has an improved mortality: 50% of children now live to be 21.

12. Which of the following test results aids in the diagnosis of cystic fibrosis?

    A. Elevated plasma protein

    B. Decreased plasma protein

    C. Elevated plasma cholesterol

    D. Elevated chloride in sweat

PART 2: CASE STUDY

Rebecca O'Shea is a 2-year-old with cystic fibrosis. Her mother is a working single parent. Rebecca was admitted to your unit with a diagnosis of pneumonia. Her mother expresses concern that Rebecca will die because working makes it difficult for her to perform the respiratory care Rebecca requires.

1. What are the major problems you would address for Rebecca during her hospital stay?

2. Your discharge plan would need to address what family needs?

3. How might community agencies be beneficial in assisting Rebecca and her mother?

■ Section Four: Inquiry and Exploration

PART 1: CRITICAL INQUIRY EXERCISES

1. In what way, if any, would you need to alter your approach and process when practicing respiratory assessment on a child compared to an adult?

2. Develop a discharge teaching plan for parents of infants or children with an upper respiratory infection.

PART 2: CRITICAL EXPLORATION EXERCISES

1. Spend a day at the cystic fibrosis clinic at a local hospital to observe follow-up care and treatment.

2. Spend a day with a respiratory therapist on a pediatric unit to observe various treatments and modalities.

Nursing Care of the Child With a Cardiovascular Disorder

CHAPTER OVERVIEW

Chapter 41 provides an overview of various cardiovascular conditions found in children. The potential effects of these conditions on the physical and psychological growth and development of the child are discussed. The use of the nursing process to plan and provide care for the client and for the family coping with a cardiovascular disorder is explored. The case study provides the student with an exercise involving preparation and management of a client undergoing a cardiac catheterization.

LEARNING OBJECTIVES

After mastering the contents of this chapter, you should be able to:

1. Describe the common cardiovascular disorders of childhood.

2. Assess a child with cardiovascular dysfunction.

3. Use the nursing process to formulate and address nursing diagnoses for the child with a cardiovascular disorder.

4. Identify National Health Goals related to cardiovascular disorders and children that nurses could be instrumental in helping the nation achieve.

5. Use critical thinking to analyze ways that nursing care of children with cardiovascular disorders could be more family-centered.

6. Synthesize knowledge of cardiovascular disorders with the nursing process to achieve quality maternal and child health nursing care.

KEY TERMS

acyanotic heart disease	hypertension
afterload	innocent heart murmur
balloon angioplasty	left-to-right shunt
cardiac catheterization	organic heart murmur
contractility	phonocardiography
cyanosis	polycythemia
cyanotic heart disease	postcardiac surgery syndrome
diastole	postperfusion syndrome
echocardiography	preload
electrocardiogram	right-to-left shunt
fluoroscopy	systole
heart failure	vasculitis

■ Section One:
Identification of Key Terms and Concepts

Match the terms in Part A with a definition or related statement from Part B. Place the letter corresponding to the answer in the space provided. (Letters may be used only once; some letters may not be used.)

PART A

1. _____ Endocarditis

2. _____ Hyperlipidemia

3. _____ Patent ductus arteriosus

4. _____ Polycythemia

5. _____ Postperfusion syndrome

6. _____ Radiography

7. _____ Atrial septal defect

8. _____ Phonocardiography

9. _____ Echocardiography

10. _____ Pulmonic stenosis

11. _____ Truncus arteriosus

12. _____ Heart failure

13. _____ Kawasaki disease

14. _____ Calcium chloride

PART B

A. Increases heart contractility; may be administered in place of epinephrine; contraindicated for patients with digitalis toxicity

B. An extreme increase in red blood cells in an attempt to increase tissue oxygenation

C. Fever, splenomegaly, general malaise, and a maculopapular rash that occurs after open heart surgery

D. Increased fatty acid level in the blood

E. Infection of the valves of the heart, generally caused by streptococci

F. Abnormal communication between the two atria where blood flows from left to right

G. Connects the pulmonary artery to the aorta; involves a left-to-right (oxygenated to unoxygenated) shunt of blood

H. Manifests a wide pulse pressure and systolic-diastolic murmur

I. Narrowing of the pulmonary valve

J. One major artery arises from the left and right ventricles

K. Results when the myocardium of the heart cannot circulate and pump enough blood to supply the tissues of the body

L. Mucocutaneous lymph node syndrome occurring almost exclusively in children before puberty

M. A diagram of heart sounds translated into electrical energy by a microphone placed on the child's chest

N. An ultrasound produced by high-frequency sound waves used to locate and study the movements and dimensions of cardiac structures

O. Furnishes an accurate picture of the heart size and contour and size of the heart chambers

■ Section Two:
Short Answer and Completion Exercises

PART 1

Complete the following fill-in-the-blank exercises.

1. In heart defects in which a connection exists between the right and left heart, the blood through the connective structure flows from _____ to _____.

2. Newborns and infants with heart disease are commonly brought to the health care facility by parents because the child is having _____ _____.

3. Chest tubes inserted in a child during open heart surgery will include an upper tube draining _____ and a lower one draining _____.

4. Rejection after cardiac transplant can occur as _____ , _____ , or _____ forms.

5. Provide the name of the cyanotic heart disease described.
   A. Includes pulmonary artery stenosis, ventricular septal defect, dextroposition of the aorta and right ventricular hypertrophy._____

   B. The aorta rises from the right ventricle instead of the left ventricle; usually accompanied by atrial and septal defects.
   _____

   C. The tricuspid valve is closed and the foramen ovale and ductus arteriosus remain patent.
   _____

6. One of the first signs of congestive heart failure in children is _____.

7. _____ _____ is an autoimmune disease that occurs as a reaction to a group A beta-hemolytic streptococcal infection.

8. Three of the five criteria for diagnosis of Kawasaki disease, other than fever, are _____ , _____ , and _____.

9. _____ _____ is the most frequent cause of cardiac arrest in children.

PART 2

Complete the following short answer exercises.

1. List the prenatal and birth information that should be discussed while obtaining a nursing history for a child with a cardiovascular disorder.

2. Relate two major areas of information to be discussed with parents taking home their child who has a heart disorder.

3. Discuss the preparatory teaching necessary for a child and family before open heart surgery.

4. Describe how innocent and organic murmurs differ relative to duration, quality, and intensity.

▪ Section Three: Critical Thinking for Application of Essential Concepts

PART 1

Circle the letter corresponding to the appropriate answer.

1. A child with coarctation of the aorta might require which of the following nursing interventions?
   A. Assisting the child and parents with coping with this terminal illness
   B. Informing females with the condition that pregnancy seldom causes problems
   C. Reassuring the child and parents that postoperative abdominal pain will subside
   D. Scheduling the surgery during early infancy to prevent complications

2. Nursing care of the child with an atrial septal defect would involve which of the following?

   A. Reporting splitting of the second heart sound immediately as a serious complication

   B. Preparing the child and family for cardiac catheterization

   C. Monitoring the diastolic murmur over the apical area that is diagnostic of the condition

   D. Teaching parents about the lifelong medications required to control the condition

3. Parents of a child with a pacemaker must be taught

   A. the procedure for cardiac defibrillation in case a dysrhythmia occurs.

   B. how to take the child's pulse accurately to determine pacemaker function.

   C. to change the pacemaker battery every year if symptoms indicate the need.

   D. that prolonged hiccuping is a harmless side effect from pacemaker leads.

4. Which of the following findings may be noted in a child with coarctation?

   A. Low blood pressure in the upper extremities

   B. High blood pressure in the lower extremities

   C. A history of headaches and nosebleeds

   D. A capillary refill of less than 5 seconds

5. Which of the following would be most effective in reducing the workload of the heart of a child with heart failure?

   A. Bed rest in a semi-Fowler's position

   B. Digoxin administration daily, IV or orally

   C. Oxygen therapy by mask, cannula, or tent

   D. Intravenous infusion of 2,000 to 3,000 mL/day

6. Which of the following is true about congestive heart failure?

   A. Edema is an early symptom of heart failure in children.

   B. Irritability and restlessness may indicate abdominal pain from hepatomegaly.

   C. Left heart failure initially presents with jugular vein distention.

   D. Right heart failure results in pulmonary edema as an initial sign.

7. Reduction of complications from rheumatic fever can be accomplished through which of the following interventions?

   A. Administration of penicillin to children with strep throat or impetigo

   B. Beginning speech therapy to reverse damage after antibiotics are completed

   C. Pushing children with chorea to perform activities requiring fine motor movement to strengthen muscles

   D. Withholding salicylates to prevent joint hemorrhage

8. Nursing interventions for a child with Kawasaki disease may include which of the following?

    A. Maintaining heavy bed coverings and clothing to keep the child warm and comfortable

    B. Palpating skin temperature and assessing capillary filling in fingers and toes

    C. Performing range-of-motion exercises to joints hourly to prevent contractures

    D. Withholding all aspirin-containing medications to prevent platelet agglutination

9. Hypertension in children most commonly

    A. manifests frequent severe symptoms.

    B. cannot be treated with diet and daily exercise.

    C. results as a secondary manifestation of another disease.

    D. will resolve before adolescence without treatment if it is primary hypertension.

PART 2

Determine if the following nursing interventions are appropriate or inappropriate.
Indicate your answer by placing an "A" or an "I" in the space provided.

1. _____ Ambulating a child immediately after a cardiac catheterization to prevent pulmonary atelectasis

2. _____ Assessing the skin surface of all black children to determine if cyanosis is present

3. _____ Loosening the dressing on the cardiac catheter site to promote comfort

4. _____ Bringing the parents of a child awaiting open heart surgery to the intensive care unit before surgery to prepare them

5. _____ Administering intravenous fluids liberally and rapidly to a child after open heart surgery to replace massive blood loss

6. _____ Reassuring the parents of a child with a ventricular septal defect that surgical repair is rarely required, even in large defects

7. _____ Preparing an infant who has just been diagnosed with pulmonic stenosis, as well as his parents, for immediate surgery

PART 3: CASE STUDY

Harriette Borders, age 5, has been complaining of headaches and fatigue. She also experienced syncope at school. She was seen at the pediatrician's office and referred to the children's hospital for a cardiac catheterization. Mr. and Mrs. Borders bring Harriette to the hospital and you are assigned to care for her during the procedure.

1. Mrs. Borders was instructed not to allow Harriette to eat or drink fluids after midnight the morning before the procedure. What was the reasoning for these instructions?

2. What is the purpose of the cardiac catheter?

3. Why is placement of the catheter in the vein necessary as part of the procedure?

4. What is the nursing responsibility regarding the vessel chosen for catheterization?

5. The child undergoing this procedure is awake during the process. It is likely that she would be anxious, afraid, and uncooperative if not prepared appropriately. What are some measures you can use to reduce Harriette's anxiety?

6. When Harriette returns from the procedure, what is the most important postoperative nursing diagnosis?

7. You inform Mr. Borders that Harriette must lie flat in bed for 3 hours after returning to her room. Explain the physiologic rationale for this statement.

■ Section Four: Inquiry and Exploration

PART 1: CRITICAL INQUIRY EXERCISES

1. Prepare a plan to teach cardiopulmonary resuscitation to family members of a child with a cardiac anomaly.

2. Prepare a teaching plan to instruct the family on how exercising and modifying nutritional intake can improve cardiovascular health. Include the National Health Goals in your plan.

3. Prepare for a class presentation an outline contrasting the hemodynamics of cyanotic and acyanotic heart disease.

PART 2: CRITICAL EXPLORATION EXERCISES

Visit a neonatal intensive care unit and assess various infants. Identify heart sounds, differences in vital signs, and feeding problems.

CHAPTER 42

Nursing Care of the Child With an Immune Disorder

CHAPTER OVERVIEW

Chapter 42 discusses the immune process as it relates to childhood illness. Immune disorders noted in childhood are reviewed. The use of the nursing process to plan and provide care for the child and the family coping with an immune disorder is explored.

LEARNING OBJECTIVES

After mastering the contents of this chapter, you should be able to:

1. Describe the immune process as it relates to childhood illness.

2. Assess the child with a disorder of the immune system.

3. Use the nursing process to formulate and address nursing diagnoses for the child with a disorder of the immune system.

4. Identify National Health Goals related to immune disorders and children that nurses could be instrumental in helping the nation achieve.

5. Identify areas related to care of the child with an immune disorder that could benefit from additional nursing research.

6. Use critical thinking to analyze ways that nursing care for the child with an immune disorder can be more family-centered.

7. Synthesize knowledge of immune disorders and the nursing process to achieve quality child health nursing care.

KEY TERMS

allergen	delayed hypersensitivity	lymphokines
anaphylaxis	environmental control	lysis
angioedema	hapten formation	macrophage
antigen	helper T cell	memory cell
autoimmunity	humoral immunity	phagocytosis
B lymphocyte	hypersensitivity response	plasma cell
cell-mediated immunity	hyposensitization	suppressor T cell
chemotaxis	immune response	T lymphocyte
complement	immunity	tolerance
contact dermatitis	immunocompetent cells	urticaria
cytotoxic response	immunogen	
cytotoxic T cells	killer T cell	

■ Section One:
Identification of Key Terms and Concepts

Match the terms in Part A with a definition or related statement from Part B. Place the letter corresponding to the answer in the space provided.

PART A

1. _____ Antigen

2. _____ Cell-mediated immunity

3. _____ Hapten

4. _____ Immunocompetent

5. _____ Immunogen

6. _____ Lymphokines

7. _____ Memory cell

8. _____ Phagocytosis

9. _____ Serum sickness

10. _____ Suppressor cells

PART B

A. The neutralization of pathogens through ingestion by white blood cells

B. An antigen that can be destroyed readily by an immune response

C. Foreign substance capable of stimulating an immune response

D. Responsible for retaining the formula or ability to produce specific immunoglobulins

E. A hypersensitivity reaction to a foreign serum antigen or drug

F. A nonantigenic substance that becomes antigenic when combined with a higher-weight molecule

G. T cells that reduce the production of immunoglobulins against a specific antigen

H. Secreted by killer cells to help prevent the migration of antigens

I. When antibodies are formed in response to a particular antigen; acquired through T-lymphocyte activity

J. Cells capable of resisting foreign invaders

■ Section Two:
Short Answer and Completion Exercises

PART 1

Complete the following fill-in-the-blank exercises.

1. _____ results from an inability to distinguish self (own tissue) from non-self (foreign tissue).

2. Congenital immunodeficiencies usually manifest after the first _____ months of life.

3. Provide the type of primary immunodeficiency for each description.

   A. Cellular immune response remains adequate; child has resistance to viral, fungal, and parasitic infections.

   _____

   B. Children are unable to respond to antigen invasion and no antibodies are produced. _____

4. Human immunodeficiency virus (HIV) is spread by two primary routes in the adult population: _____ contact and _____ contact.

5. Universal precautions entail the use of _____ when physical contact with bodily secretions is likely.

6. Assessment of the exact symptoms of an allergy is important in helping to identify the _____.

7. The three goals for therapy in childhood allergy situations are to _____ , _____ , and _____.

8. The best way to identify the specific allergies in a child with food allergies is the use of a _____ _____ or an elimination diet.

9. When a child is stung by a bee, the immediate action should be to apply _____ to the site to minimize the absorption of the venom.

PART 2

Complete the following short answer exercises.

1. State two measures a parent can take to decrease allergies in the bedroom, living room, and at school.

   _____   _____

2. Compare seborrheic dermatitis and infantile eczema relative to the presence of itching, age of onset, length of disease, and mood of the child.

3. Differentiate between congenital and acquired immunodeficiency disorders.

4. Discuss the purpose and use of skin testing when assessing allergies in children.

■ Section Three: Critical Thinking for Application of Essential Concepts

PART 1

Circle the letter corresponding to the appropriate answer.

1. Nurses can help the nation achieve health goals related to human immunodeficiency virus by doing which of the following?
    A. Instructing young people that IV drugs are safer than oral drugs, although both are bad
    B. Encouraging drug addicts to share needles with friends only, if they must use drugs
    C. Educating children about the importance of using condoms or practicing abstinence
    D. Avoiding discussions related to sex around adolescents younger than 18 years old

2. Janice has a deficiency that affects her humoral immunity. This means she may have inadequate
    A. B cells.
    B. antigens.
    C. T cells.
    D. allergens.

3. Which of the following is **not** an atopic disorder?
    A. Asthma
    B. Hay fever
    C. Atopic dermatitis
    D. Serum sickness

4. Which of the following actions would be appropriate when providing care to a child with a hypersensitivity condition?
    A. Having a syringe filled with a 1:5 dilution of the antigen on hand to counteract an unexpected anaphylactic reaction from skin testing
    B. Keeping the child at the health care setting for 30 minutes after the hyposensitization process
    C. Excluding the child with allergies from planning methods of environmental control to avoid resistance to the changes
    D. Encouraging parents who know of familial allergy patterns to bottle-feed infants

PART 2

Determine if the following nursing interventions are appropriate or inappropriate. Indicate your answer by placing an "A" or an "I" in the space provided.

1. _____ A child who faints after an insect bite or drug injection should be assessed and treated, if indicated, for anaphylaxis.

2. _____ Administer a smaller-than-normal dosage of foreign serum to a child known to manifest serum sickness.

3. _____ Children who develop urticaria as a result of exposure to extreme temperatures should not be allowed to swim in cold water.

4. _____ Instruct parents of children with atopic dermatitis to cover the area with dressings coated in Burow's solution.

PART 3: CASE STUDY

José is a 4-year-old with a primary B cell, IgA type immune deficiency disorder. He is admitted to your unit with an upper respiratory tract infection. His parents are concerned that his brothers and sisters will also contract the immune deficiency, so they won't let their other children play with José.

1. What is the most important concept you must include in a teaching plan for José's parents?

2. How would you approach his parents regarding their fears about José's siblings?

3. What concerns would you have about caring for José?

■ Section Four: Inquiry and Exploration

PART 1: CRITICAL INQUIRY EXERCISES

1. Prepare a teaching plan on the diagnosis of allergic rhinitis for a child and his or her family.

2. What would your response be to a fellow nurse who refuses to care for a client with contact dermatitis because the nurse fears becoming infected?

PART 2: CRITICAL EXPLORATION EXERCISES

During a clinical experience, monitor care provided to a client with AIDS. Note the precautions used in care and the client's emotional response to the care and care providers. Note the care that you felt was particularly good, as well as ways in which care-physical and emotional-might have been improved.

Nursing Care of the Child With an Infectious Disorder

CHAPTER OVERVIEW

Chapter 43 discusses common infectious disorders of childhood. The nursing techniques required to address the needs of children and their families when coping with an infectious disease are reviewed. The use of the nursing process to plan and provide care for the child with an infectious disease and his or her family is explored.

LEARNING OBJECTIVES

After mastering the contents of this chapter, you should be able to:

1. Describe the causes and course of common infectious disorders of childhood.

2. Assess the child with an infection.

3. Use the nursing process to identify and address nursing diagnoses related to infection in children.

4. Identify National Health Goals related to infectious disorders and children that nurses could be instrumental in helping the nation achieve.

5. Identify areas of nursing care related to children with infectious diseases that could benefit from additional nursing research.

6. Use critical thinking to analyze ways that care of the child with an infection can be more family-centered.

7. Synthesize knowledge of infectious diseases and the nursing process to achieve quality child health nursing care.

KEY TERMS

catarrhal stage	Koplik's spots
chain of infection	means of transmission
complement	portal of entry
convalescent period	portal of exit
enanthem	prodromal period
exanthem	reservoir
exotoxin	septicemia
fomites	susceptible host
incubation period	toxoid
interferon	

■ Section One:
Identification of Key Terms and Concepts

PART 1

Indicate if the following statements are true or false by placing a "T" or "F" in the space provided.

1. __F__ Roseola infantum is a herpes viral infection.

2. __T__ Rubella occurs primarily during the spring in older school-age children.

3. __T__ Rubeola has a 10- to 11-day prodromal period and is referred to as 7-day measles.

4. __T__ Rubeola has a rash that turns from brown to red and always fades on pressure.

5. __T__ Varicella is highly contagious and can be spread by direct or indirect contact of saliva or vesicles.

6. __T__ Herpes zoster occurs upon second and subsequent exposure to the varicella-zoster virus of chicken pox.

7. __F__ The echoviruses are responsible for herpangina, a condition affecting the child's oral cavity.

8. __T__ Poliovirus infections are transmitted most easily when the virus is present in the gastrointestinal tract.

9. __F__ The paralysis resulting from the poliovirus is generally symmetrical, with the child's arms being affected most commonly.

10. __T__ Herpes simplex virus remains latent in a child's body, so the child becomes a permanent carrier.

PART 2

Match each term in Part A with its definition or related statement in Part B. Place the letter corresponding to the answer in the space provided. (Letters may be used only once; some letters may not be used.)

PART A

1. __B__ Pathogens

2. __C__ Prodromal period

3. __E__ Chain of infection

4. __F__ Reservoir

5. __G__ Fomites

6. __I__ Herpes labialis

7. __A__ Exanthem

8. __D__ Illness

9. __J__ Interferon ✓

10. __K__ Furuncle ✓   10/10

PART B

A. A rash on the skin

B. Organisms that cause disease in children

C. A time between the beginning of nonspecific symptoms and specific symptoms

D. The stage during which specific symptoms are evident

E. The method by which organisms spread and enter a new individual to cause disease

F. The container or place in which organisms grow and reproduce

G. Inanimate objects such as soil, food, or water

H. Living carriers such as insects

I. A cold sore, representing a type 1 herpesvirus invasion

J. A lymphokine; prevents cells from being host to more than one virus at a time

K. An infection of the hair follicle; a boil

■ Section Two: Short Answer and Completion Exercises

PART 1

Complete the following fill-in-the-blank exercises.

1. __incubation__ is the time between the invasion of an organism and the onset of symptoms of infection.

2. The sources of pathogens are classified as __viruses__ , __bacteria__ , __fungi__ , __rickettsia__ , and __helminths__ .

3. __Rocky Mountain spotted fever__ is a common rickettsial disease transmitted by a tick.

4. __hookworm__ enters the body through the skin, migrates to the intestinal tract, and thrives on blood, causing severe anemia.

5. __Chicken pox (varicella)__ is highly contagious and spreads by direct or indirect contact of saliva or vesicles.

6. __Warts__ represents one of the most common dermatologic diseases in children.

7. Once the rabies disease process begins, rabies is invariably __fatal__ .

8. The incubation period for mumps is __14__ to __21__ days, and the period of communicability is shortly before or after the onset of __parotitis__ .

9. A serious complication from mumps occurring in males over the age of puberty is __orchitis__ .

PART 2

Determine the type of precaution needed for each of the isolation situations listed below. Indicate your answer by placing one or more of the following abbreviations in the space provided: "Pr" = private room; "G" = gown; "Gl" = glove; "M" = mask.

1. _Pr, G, Gl, M_ Respiratory isolation ✓

2. _____ Enteric precautions Pr, Gl, G

3. _____ Drainage secretion precautions Gl, mx   (Gl & G)

4. _____ Contact isolation Pr, G, Gl, M

5. _____ Strict isolation "Pr, G, Gl, M " ✓

PART 3

Complete the following short answer exercises.

1. Discuss the method through which organisms are spread, listing the elements necessary to complete the chain of infection.

   - direct/indirect contact, inhalation, ingestion, abrasion, burns, wounds

2. Discuss circumstances that cause a child to be susceptible to infection.

3. Discuss why a child should be skin tested for tuberculosis before measles vaccination.

4. Describe the universal precautions health care providers should take in all clinical settings.

5. List the signs and symptoms of scarlet fever.

▪ Section Three:
Critical Thinking for Application of Essential Concepts

PART 1

Circle the letter corresponding to the appropriate answer.

1. Belinda, age 6, has been diagnosed with infectious mononucleosis. The nurse should do which of the following?

    A. Encourage Belinda to return to school and normal physical activity after 10 days.

    B. Limit Belinda's fluids to decrease the workload of the spleen.

    C. Keep Belinda in bed for a week or more with quiet games and books.

    D. Push on Belinda's upper stomach daily and report any complaints of tenderness.

2. When a child is scratched by a cat, the parents should be instructed to do which of the following?

    A. Destroy the animal to prevent subsequent attacks.

    B. Submit the animal for a blood test to aid in the diagnosis of cat scratch disease.

    C. Monitor the child for irritability and changes in level of consciousness.

    D. Place ice on enlarged nodes to control and decrease swelling.

3. To prevent exposure to Lyme disease, an individual should do which of the following?

    A. Wear dark-colored clothing to avoid attracting ticks.

    B. Inspect the skin of children exposed to wooded areas for tick bites.

    C. Apply calamine lotion to tick bite areas immediately to remove poison.

    D. If a tick is noted on the skin, remove it quickly using your fingernails.

PART 2

Determine if the following nursing interventions are appropriate or inappropriate.
Indicate your answer by placing an "A" or an "I" in the space provided.

1. 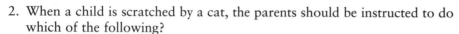 Instruct parents to wash impetigo skin crusts daily with half-strength peroxide.

2. _A_ Assess for hypersensitivity to iodine or shellfish before administering the antitoxin to a child with diphtheria.

3. _A_ Explain to parents that the child with pertussis (whooping cough) must be watched closely for airway obstruction.

4. _A_ Monitor the client suspected of exposure to tetanus for redness and pus at the site of entrance of the bacillus.

5. _A_ Inform parents that a temperature of 101° to 102°F is an expected symptom in children with tetanus.

6. _A_ Instruct parents to monitor children with possible tick bites for signs and symptoms of Rocky Mountain spotted fever.

✓ 7. __I__ Teach parents of children with pet birds that if the bird doesn't appear ill, the child cannot contract psittacosis.

✓ 8. __A__ Instruct parents of school-age children with head lice that lice infestation can occur regardless of personal hygiene.

✗ 9. __A__ Wash the skin of a patient who has scabies with warm soapy water daily to destroy the mites.

✗ 10. __I__ Examine a child's anal area to detect the presence of pinworms.

PART 3: CASE STUDY

Petro Juan, age 17, is admitted to your unit with infectious mononucleosis. Petro is complaining of tiredness but his parents are encouraging him to be more active to regain his strength.

1. What are some factors that contributed to Petro being a susceptible (at risk) host for infection?

2. What would be your response to Petro's parents regarding their approach to Petro's treatment?

3. What factors should be included in the nutritional plan of care?

■ Section Four: Inquiry and Exploration

PART 1: CRITICAL INQUIRY EXERCISES

1. If your patient was on strict isolation and you observed another health care professional entering the patient's room without wearing protective items, what would you do?

2. A patient is admitted to your unit, and you suspect from his history that he has had a recent exposure to a person with an active case of varicella. Your hospital requires a physician's order before placing a patient on respiratory isolation. What actions would you take?

PART 2: CRITICAL EXPLORATION EXERCISES

While on a clinical unit, provide care for a child on various types of isolation (e.g., respiratory, enteric). Compare precautions taken with each patient when: emptying urine, providing the bedpan, or collecting and testing a blood specimen.

CHAPTER 44

Nursing Care of the Child With a Hematologic Disorder

CHAPTER OVERVIEW

The disease process of some blood disorders in children may be insidious; presenting symptoms in the early stage of the disease may not alert parents. However, many of these illnesses can become life-threatening. The nurse must be able to synthesize knowledge of findings from systems assessments with the signs and symptoms of hematologic disorders. Chapter 44 provides the student with the knowledge to care for the child and family with a hematologic disorder. The case study involves the altered hematologic processes in a sickle cell crisis.

LEARNING OBJECTIVES

After mastering the contents of this chapter, you should be able to:

1. Describe the major hematologic disorders of childhood, such as sickle cell anemia, iron-deficiency anemia, hemophilia, and thalassemia.

2. Assess the child with a hematologic disorder.

3. Use the nursing process to identify and address nursing diagnoses for the child with a hematologic disorder.

4. Identify National Health Goals related to children with hematologic disorders that nurses could be instrumental in helping the nation achieve.

5. Use critical thinking to analyze ways that nursing care for a child with a hematologic disorder could be more family-centered.

6. Synthesize knowledge of hematologic disorders in children with the nursing process to achieve quality child health nursing care.

KEY TERMS

agranulocytes
allogeneic transplantation
aplastic anemias
autologous transplantation
blood dyscrasias
blood plasma
direct bilirubin
erythroblasts
erythrocytes
erythropoietin
granulocytes
Heinz bodies

hemochromatosis
hemoglobin
hemolysis
hemosiderosis
hypodermoclysis
leukocytess
leukopenia
megakaryocytes
normoblasts
pancytopenia
petechiae

plethora
poikilocytic
polycythemia
priapism
purpura
reticulocytes
sickle cell crisis
sickle cell trait
synergeneic transplantation
thrombocytes
thrombocytopenia

■ Section One:
Identification of Key Terms and Concepts

Match the terms in Part A with a definition or related statement from Part B. Place the letter corresponding to the answer in the space provided.

PART A

1. _____ Heinz bodies

2. _____ Leukopenia

3. _____ Disseminated intravascular coagulation

4. _____ Plethora

5. _____ Allogeneic transplantation

6. _____ Purpura

7. _____ Normochromic anemia

8. _____ Hypochromic anemia

9. _____ Erythropoietin

10. _____ Poikilocytic

PART B

A. Acquired disorder of blood clotting that results from excessive trauma

B. Involves the transfer of bone marrow from an immune-compatible donor and its intravenous infusion to the recipient

C. Odd-shaped particles in red blood cells

D. Impaired production of erythrocytes by the bone marrow or loss of circulatory red blood cells

E. Marked reddened appearance of the skin

F. Red blood cells that are irregular in shape

G. Results from a reduced number of white blood cells

H. A hormone produced by the kidneys that stimulates the formation of red blood cells

I. Hemorrhagic rash or small hemorrhages occurring in the superficial layer of the skin

J. Reduction in the diameter of cells when hemoglobin synthesis is inadequate

■ Section One:
Short Answer and Completion Exercises

PART 1

Complete the following fill-in-the-blank exercises.

1. _____ are round nonnucleated bodies formed by bone marrow; normal range in count is 150,000 to 300,000/cm.

2. _____ _____ _____ is a procedure involving intravenous infusion for children with acquired aplastic anemia.

3. _____ is excessive destruction of red blood cells.

4. _____ are vehicles used to transport oxygen to and carry carbon dioxide away from body cells.

5. _____ __ _____ _____ is a potentially lethal immunologic response of donor T cells against the tissue of the recipient.

PART 2

Complete the following short answer questions.

1. Describe how congenital aplastic anemia differs from acquired aplastic anemia.

2. Why is it appropriate to administer two infusions concurrently when administering a long-term packed red cell infusion program?

■ Section Three: Critical Thinking for Application of Essential Concepts

PART 1

Circle the letter corresponding to the appropriate answer.

1. Which of the following foods supplies the better source of iron for the infant?
   A. Human breast milk
   B. Iron-fortified cereals
   C. Vegetables
   D. Fruit

2. Which of the following drugs is contraindicated for a child who is diagnosed as deficient in glucose 6-phosphate dehydrogenase (G-6PD)?
   A. Acetylsalicylic acid
   B. Acetaminophen
   C. Ampicillin
   D. Tetracycline

3. Mrs. Hill brings her 10-month-old son, Keith, to the emergency room with a temperature of 104.6°F. He is dehydrated and has edema of the right ankle. He is admitted to the pediatric ward. The assessment revealed a diagnosis of sickle cell anemia. The clinical manifestations of sickle cell crisis are a result of a(n):

    A. pain in the joints of the hands.

    B. amino acid deficiency.

    C. inborn error of metabolism.

    D. stasis of abnormal red blood cells in vessels.

4. Which of the following might be a finding indicating sickle cell crisis in Keith?

    A. Elevated serum sodium

    B. Dry mucous membranes

    C. Loss of appetite

    D. Hematuria and flank pain

5. Keith's anemia has not manifested before this age because in the first few months of his life there existed

    A. increased immunity protection from maternal antibodies.

    B. immature liver functioning.

    C. fetal hemoglobin.

    D. increased circulatory blood volumes.

PART 2: CASE STUDY

Phyllis, age 12, has been experiencing problems from sickle cell anemia since she was 1 year old. She has been admitted to the pediatric ward of a children's hospital with an admitting diagnosis of sickle cell crisis.

1. Since Phyllis has previously been diagnosed with sickle cell anemia, what characteristics would the physician most probably find on this admission?

2. What are the primary nursing goals when caring for Phyllis?

3. What precautionary measures are there to consider when administering IV fluids to Phyllis?

4. What findings on the assessment would suggest that Phyllis needs oxygen supplementation?

▪ Section Four: Inquiry and Exploration

PART 1: CRITICAL INQUIRY EXERCISES

1. Develop a nursing care plan that addresses the nursing process to care for the patient with aplastic anemia.

2. Create a list of foods that would be most appropriate for a school-age child with iron-deficiency anemia.

PART 2: CRITICAL EXPLORATION EXERCISES

Attend a camp for children with sickle cell anemia. Assess the program's objectives and goals for camp participants.

Nursing Care of the Child With a Gastrointestinal Disorder

CHAPTER OVERVIEW

Chapter 45 describes the child with a disorder of the gastrointestinal system. The chapter addresses the importance of the gastrointestinal system to the entire body's ability to grow and develop in a healthy manner.

LEARNING OBJECTIVES

After mastering the contents of this chapter, you should be able to:

1. Describe common gastrointestinal disorders in children, such as vomiting, diarrhea, and appendicitis.

2. Assess the child with a gastrointestinal disorder.

3. Formulate nursing diagnoses for the child with a gastrointestinal disorder.

4. Develop outcomes for the child with a gastrointestinal disorder.

5. Plan nursing care with specific goals for the child with a gastrointestinal disorder

6. Implement nursing care for the child with a gastrointestinal disorder.

7. Evaluate outcomes for effectiveness and achievement of care.

8. Identify National Health Goals related to gastrointestinal disorders and children that nurses could be instrumental in helping the nation achieve.

9. Identify areas of care related to gastrointestinal disorders and children that could benefit from additional nursing research or application of evidence-based practice.

10. Analyze ways that nursing care of the child with a gastrointestinal disorder can be more family-centered

11. Integrate knowledge of gastrointestinal disorders with the nursing process to achieve quality maternal and child health nursing care.

KEY TERMS

aganglionic megacolon	inguinal hernia	necrotizing enterocolitis
anion	insensible loss	nutritional marasmus
appendicitis	intussusception	overhydration
beriberi	irritable bowel syndrome	pellagra
celiac disease	isotonic dehydration	peptic ulcer
chalasia	keratomalacia	pyloric stenosis
Crohn's disease	kwashiorkor	rickets
dehydration	liver transplantation	steatorrhea
gastroesophageal reflux	McBurney's point	ulcerative colitis
hepatitis	Meckel's diverticulum	volvulus
hiatal hernia	metabolic acidosis	xerophthalmia

■ Section One:
Identification of Key Terms and Concepts

Match the terms in Part A with a definition or related statement from Part B. Place the letter corresponding to the answer in the space provided. (Letters may be used only once; some letters may not be used.)

PART A

1. __G__ Achalasia — C / B

2. __C__ Ganglionic megacolon

3. __H__ Hiatal hernia B

4. __A__ Isotonic dehydration

5. __D__ Kwashiorkor

6. __E__ Marasmus

31 6 (A)

PART B

A. Loss of body water and salt in proportion to each other

B. Hirschsprung's disease, the absence of nerve cells and peristaltic waves in a section of the bowel

C. Gastroesophageal reflux due to a neuromuscular disturbance that causes a lax cardiac sphincter and lower esophagus

D. A disease caused by protein deficiency seen more frequently in children ages 1 to 3 years

E. A disease caused by deficiency of all food groups

F. Loss of body water out of proportion to salt

G. Intermittent protrusion of the stomach through the esophageal opening in the diaphragm

H. Protrusion of a section of the bowel into the inguinal ring

■ Section Two:
Short Answer and Completion Exercises

PART 1

Complete the following short answer exercises.

1. List five symptoms and lab findings of metabolic alkalosis.

_____   _____

_____   _____

_____

2. List three questions that must be asked when taking a history of vomiting that would help differentiate it from regurgitation.

_____

_____

_____

3. List the glands that secrete saliva.

parotid, sublingual, submandibular

4. List six symptoms of dehydration.

sunken eyes   *Poor Skin turgor*

pale skin   _____

lethargic   _____

5. Describe the findings seen on assessment of the child with intussusception.

6. Describe the pathophysiologic process that occurs with celiac disease.

PART 2

Complete the following fill-in-the-blank exercises.

1. The nurse is counseling Mrs. Anderson about her 8-month-old baby girl, Adrienne. Adrienne has been "spitting up" food after her feedings. The problem started about 3 weeks ago. The physician tells the nurse that Adrienne has chalasia. Chalasia is ~~gastr~~ *GER* ____.

2. The "spitting up" associated with chalasia is described as *effortless* and *non projectile*.

3. Chalasia is usually self-limiting as the esophageal sphincter matures. However, if not treated, more serious problems might develop, such as *dehydr,* or *alkalosis*.

4. Some good advice for Mrs. Anderson would be that she use a *thicker* formula.

■ Section Three:
Critical Thinking for Application of Essential Concepts

PART 1

Circle the letter corresponding to the appropriate answer.

1. The severity of dehydration is measured by the percentage of weight loss. If a child weighed 15 lb and has lost 0.8 kg, what is the classification of his dehydration?

   A. Mild

   B. Moderate

   C. Severe

   D. Scant

   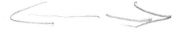

2. A patient's lab values are urine pH 5, bicarb 14, serum pH 7.24. These values would indicate

   A. metabolic acidosis.

   B. metabolic alkalosis.

   C. a history of vomiting.

   D. an excessive loss of chloride ion.

3. Which of the following nursing interventions might allay any guilt felt by the parents of a child with achalasia? GER

   A. Suggest the parents step outside the room while you feed the child so they do not view the "spitting up."

   B. Offer suggestions in positioning, since success through this measure builds confidence.

   C. Tell the parents that they were preparing the formula wrong and that this caused the condition.

   D. Reassure parents that this condition is usually due to dysentery and is not their fault.

PART 2: CASE STUDY

Aaron is 8 months old. His birth was uneventful and he has exhibited no previous health problems. Today his mother brings him to the emergency room exhibiting symptoms of dehydration.

1. What should be the normal fluid intake and output for Aaron?

2. What are the major sources and minor sources of fluid loss for infants?

3. What are the major history and physical assessments you would make for Aaron?

■ Section Four: Inquiry and Exploration

PART 1: CRITICAL INQUIRY EXERCISES

1. Create a teaching plan for the parents of a child with pyloric stenosis. Include preparation for hospitalization, surgery, and the recovery period.

2. Describe a process for determining if a patient's dehydration is isotonic, hypotonic, or hypertonic.

PART 2: CRITICAL EXPLORATION EXERCISES

Visit a day-care center. Ask what the rules are regarding care of the child with diarrhea, fever, or vomiting. Observe the staff as they implement the infection control guidelines, and determine if these techniques are sufficient.

Nursing Care of the Child With a Renal or Urinary Tract Disorder

CHAPTER OVERVIEW

Chapter 46 discusses common renal and urinary tract disorders that occur in children and the nursing care needed for these children and their families. The normal function of the renal system is reviewed. The use of the nursing process to plan and provide care for the child and family with a renal or urinary tract disorder is explored.

LEARNING OBJECTIVES

After mastering the contents of this chapter, you should be able to:

1. Describe common renal and urinary disorders that occur in children, such as urinary tract infection (UTI), nephrosis, and glomerulonephritis.

2. Assess a child for a renal or urinary tract disorder.

3. Use the nursing process to identify and address nursing diagnoses related to renal or urinary disorders.

4. Identify National Health Goals related to renal or urinary tract disorders and children that nurses can be instrumental in helping the nation achieve.

5. Use critical thinking to analyze methods for making nursing care of the child with a renal or urinary disorder more family-centered.

6. Synthesize knowledge of renal and urinary tract disorders with the nursing process to achieve quality child health nursing care.

KEY TERMS

acute transplant rejection
Alport's syndrome
azotemia
Bowman's capsule
dialysis
enuresis
epispadias
exstrophy of the bladder
glomerular filtration rate

glomerulonephritis
hydronephrosis
hypospadias
nephrosis
patent urachus
polycystic kidney
postural proteinuria
prune belly syndrome
vesicoureteral reflux

■ Section One:
Identification of Key Terms and Concepts

Match the terms in Part A with a definition or related statement from Part B. Place the letter corresponding to the answer in the space provided.

PART A

1. _____ Prune belly syndrome

2. _____ Azotemia

3. _____ Cystoscopy

4. _____ Cryptorchidism

5. _____ Enuresis

6. _____ Hypospadias

7. _____ Histocompatibility

8. _____ Acute transplant rejection

9. _____ Alport's syndrome

10. _____ Patent urachus

PART B

A. An autosomal dominant inherited disorder with chronic renal failure

B. A fistula between the bladder and the umbilicus

C. The opening of the urethra onto the ventral or lower surface of the penis

D. Direct viewing of the bladder or ureter openings for examination

E. Undescended testes often noted with hypospadias

F. Involuntary voiding past the age when a child is expected to have attained bladder control

G. Rejection that develops within 3 months following transplant

H. Urethral obstruction in utero from abnormal urethral valves

I. Exists when two people have like human leukocyte antigen (HLA) agglutinins

J. The accumulation of nitrogen waste in the bloodstream, often due to oliguria

■ Section Two:
Short Answer and Completion Exercises

PART 1

Complete the following fill-in-the-blank exercises.

1. An increase in blood levels of the products of cell metabolism such as

   _____ may indicate poor kidney function.

2. _____ is a retrograde flow of urine from the bladder to the ureters that

   may lead to a urinary tract infection.

3. _____ kidney is a condition involving abnormal development of the collecting tubules in which fluid-filled cysts, instead of kidney tissue, form in utero; it may be unilateral or bilateral.

4. Glomerulonephritis involves the obstruction of the glomeruli due to complement fixation activated by an _____-_____ reaction, stimulated most often by a streptococcal infection.

5. The four characteristic symptoms of nephrotic syndrome are _____ , _____ , _____ , and _____ .

6. Children with hemolytic-uremic syndrome usually have _____ skin coloring as well as the major symptoms of _____ with proteinuria, _____ , and urinary casts in urine.

PART 2

Complete the following short answer exercises.

1. Explain why girls are at higher risk for urinary tract infections than boys.

2. Differentiate between primary and secondary enuresis, and provide one possible physiologic and one psychological cause for secondary enuresis.

3. Compare and contrast the symptoms and treatment for nephrotic syndrome and acute glomerulonephritis.

4. Discuss the primary difference in the etiology of acute and chronic renal failure.

5. Discuss the dietary restriction of salt in a child with chronic renal failure.

■ Section Three:
Critical Thinking for Application of Essential Concepts

PART 1

Circle the letter corresponding to the appropriate answer.

1. Which of the following interventions might be most effective in preventing glomerulonephritis?

   A. Daily administration of children's multivitamins and iron

   B. Increasing all children's fluid intake to 3 liters daily

   C. Prompt evaluation of childhood complaints of sore throat

   D. Teaching children to void promptly when the urge is felt

2. Which of the following would most likely be noted in a child with acute glomerulonephritis?

   A. Blood pressure of 90/40

   B. Hypovolemia and signs of dehydration

   C. Hematuria and pulmonary edema

   D. Severe, foul-smelling diarrhea

3. The nurse could implement which of the following measures for a child who demonstrated enuresis with no apparent organic cause?

   A. Encourage the child to discuss concerns relative to the birth of a new sibling or other problems.

   B. Instruct the parents never to let the child drink after dinner.

   C. Limit the fluids of children with sickle cell anemia since they are most prone to this condition.

   D. Teach parents to strictly enforce bladder training with the child.

4. Bobby, age 10, has a diagnosis of acute nephrotic syndrome. Which of the following nursing interventions would be most appropriate?

   A. Administering liberal IV and oral fluids to offset the accompanying dehydration

   B. Discussing the cushingoid effects of prednisone therapy with the child and parents

   C. Reassuring the child and parents that diuretics will quickly reduce the edema

   D. Preparing the child and parents for the frequently terminal outcome of the disease

5. Which of the following would be an appropriate explanation to provide to the parents of a child with severe hypertension awaiting a renal transplant?

   A. After the child's nonfunctioning kidneys are removed, the child will have no food restrictions.

   B. Removal of only one kidney is necessary to provide room for the new kidney.

   C. Reluctant younger siblings can still serve as a kidney donor as long as the parent signs both surgery consent forms.

   D. The transplanted kidney will be placed in the abdomen, not in the usual kidney space.

PART 2

Determine if the following nursing interventions are appropriate or inappropriate.
Indicate your answer by placing an "A" or an "I" in the space provided.

1. _____ Position an infant with exstrophy of the bladder on his back to facilitate the bladder's storage capacity.

2. _____ Place a child with exstrophy of the bladder in a tub bath daily to remove sediment and maintain good hygiene.

3. _____ Stress the importance of the repair of hypospadias before the child's maturity to prevent fertility problems.

4. _____ Prepare children with urinary tract infections for diagnostic procedures to rule out urethral stenosis or bladder reflux.

5. _____ Teach girls to wipe from back to front after voiding or stooling.

6. _____ Encourage a child with a urinary tract infection to drink liberal amounts of fluids.

7. _____ Instruct women who are prone to "honeymoon cystitis" to void before coitus to decrease the incidence of infection.

8. _____ Instruct children and parents, after ureteral reflux surgery, to save small samples of voidings for a period of time.

9. _____ Place a child in a warm tub bath during the period immediately after ureteral reflux surgery to facilitate bladder emptying.

10. _____ Administer Kayexalate to a child with acute renal failure whose serum potassium is 3.0.

11. _____ Instruct the parents of a child with chronic renal failure in the preparation of a diet low in protein and phosphorus.

12. _____ Administer aluminum hydroxide, alternating with milk, to children with chronic renal failure to prevent ulcer formation.

13. _____ Encourage children receiving corticosteroids to discuss angry feelings regarding their change in appearance.

14. _____ Inform children undergoing peritoneal dialysis that their blood is being cleaned by rinsing it outside their body.

15. _____ Monitor children undergoing hemodialysis frequently during the procedure to detect changes in cerebral tissue perfusion.

PART 3: CASE STUDY

Rebecca, age 2, is admitted to your unit with dehydration and acute strep throat. After 3 days of treatment and IV fluids, you notice that Rebecca's urine output has remained low and her blood levels of nitrogen and creatinine are elevated.

1. What type of renal failure has Rebecca probably developed? What other symptoms of renal failure might you notice?

2. How would you explain Rebecca's renal condition to her parents?

3. What activity level would you expect to be ordered for Rebecca, and how would you help her maintain it?

■ Section Four: Inquiry and Exploration

PART 1: CRITICAL INQUIRY EXERCISES

1. Prepare a teaching plan for a child discharged on continuous ambulatory peritoneal dialysis.

2. Your patient, admitted after an automobile accident, has just been diagnosed as being brain dead. What would your response be if the doctor asked you to approach the family regarding donating the patient's kidneys? When and how would you choose to approach the family?

PART 2: CRITICAL EXPLORATION EXERCISES

Visit a dialysis unit; review three or four charts and note the various causes of renal failure.

CHAPTER 47

Nursing Care of the Child With a Reproductive Disorder

CHAPTER OVERVIEW

Reproductive disorders in children range from mild infection to serious anatomic malformations. All require prompt treatment to prevent later disruption in sexual or reproductive health. Sensitive and careful questioning when assessing children with reproductive system dysfunction is essential. This chapter addresses the illnesses affecting external reproductive structures and reproductive organs. The case study affords the student the opportunity to plan the nursing care for an adolescent with an altered assessment of the male reproductive system.

LEARNING OBJECTIVES

After mastering the contents of this chapter, you should be able to:

1. Describe common reproductive disorders in children.

2. Assess the child with a reproductive disorder.

3. Use the nursing process to identify and address nursing diagnoses related to a child's reproductive illness.

4. Identify National Health Goals related to reproductive disorders and children that nurses can be instrumental in helping the nation achieve.

5. Identify areas related to care of children with reproductive disorders that could benefit from additional nursing research.

6. Use critical thinking to analyze ways that nursing care for the child with a reproductive disorder can be more family-centered.

7. Synthesize knowledge of reproductive disorders in children with the nursing process to achieve quality child health nursing care.

KEY TERMS

amenorrhea
anovulatory
cryptorchidism
dysmenorrhea
endometriosis
fibrocystic breast disease
gynecomastia
hermaphrodite
hydrocele
menorrhagia
metrorrhagia

mittelschmerz
orchiectomy
orchiopexy
pelvic inflammatory disease
premenstrual syndrome (PMS)
pseudohermaphrodite
sexually transmitted disease (STD)
toxic shock syndrome
varicocele
vulvovaginitis

■ Section One:
Identification of Key Terms and Concepts

Match the terms in Part A with a definition or related statement from Part B. Place the letter corresponding to the answer in the space provided. (Letters may be used only once; some letters will not be used.)

PART A

1. _____ Hymen

2. _____ Amenorrhea

3. _____ Balanoposthitis

4. _____ Hydrocele

5. _____ Metrorrhagia

6. _____ Orchiectomy

7. _____ Pseudohermaphrodite

8. _____ Toxic shock syndrome

9. _____ Imperforate hymen

10. _____ Pelvic inflammatory disease

PART B

A. An abnormally heavy menstrual flow

B. Removal of the testes

C. Inflammation of the glans and prepuce of the penis

D. Infant with some external features of both sexes, although only ovaries or testes are present

E. Most frequently caused by gonorrheal infections or chlamydia

F. Membranous ring of tissue blocking the vaginal opening

G. An infection caused by toxin-producing strains of staphylococcus

H. Fluid collected in the space called the processus vaginalis

I. A membranous ring of tissue totally occluding the vagina

J. Absence of menstrual flow; may suggest pregnancy

K. Bleeding between menstrual periods

■ Section Two:
Short Answer and Completion Exercises

PART 1

Complete the following fill-in-the-blank exercises.

1. A _____ is abnormal dilation of the veins of the spermatic cord.

2. _____ is an enlargement of the male breast.

3. Testicular cancer has symptoms of heaviness of the _____. It is
   _____ and _____ rapidly.

4. _____ is defined as experiencing abdominal pain during ovulation. The
   discomfort is felt on either side of the _____ , near an ovary.

5. _____ is an inflammation of the glans and prepuce of the penis.

6. _____ is failure of both testes to descend from the abdominal cavity to
   the scrotum.

PART 2

Complete the following short answer exercises.

1. Define ambiguous genitalia.

2. List the four anatomic structures involved in pelvic inflammatory disease.

   _____   _____

   _____   _____

3. What are three theories on the causes of premenstrual syndrome (PMS)?

   _____   _____

   _____

4. What information on the reproductive life cycle should be included when
   educating the patient who has experienced pelvic inflammatory disease?

■ Section Three:
Critical Thinking for Application of Essential Concepts

PART 1

Circle the letter corresponding to the appropriate answer.

1. Baby J, 1 day old, is born with ambiguous genitalia. The nurse would incorporate teaching to help the parents as their child undergoes which of the following tests to determine gender?

   A. Blood cultures

   B. Colposcopy

   C. Karyotyping

   D. Sedimentation rate

2. A young female who has trichomonas vaginalis may experience which of the following symptoms?

   A. Greenish vaginal discharge

   B. Cream cheese-like vaginal discharge

   C. Patchy white lesions on vaginal wall

   D. Frothy white or grayish-green vaginal discharge

3. Which of the following is a symptom of the final stage of syphilis?

   A. Blindness

   B. Chancre

   C. Low-grade fever

   D. Lymphadenopathy

4. Fibrocystic breast disease is the most common benign breast disease among women. The therapeutic interventions to reduce discomfort include all of the following except

   A. acetaminophen.

   B. oral contraceptives.

   C. caffeine.

   D. Danocrine.

5. The most common source of introduction of the organism causing toxic shock syndrome is

   A. deep buccal tissue.

   B. vaginal wall tissue.

   C. urethral meatus.

   D. nasal mucous membranes.

PART 2: CASE STUDY

Peter, age 14, is seen in your clinic. He states he had sex with a girl who recently told him she was diagnosed with syphilis. He insists that nobody else know about his visit to the clinic since he can pay for the medicine himself.

1. What symptoms would you question Peter about, and what diagnostic procedures would you prepare him for?

2. What information would you include in your teaching plan for Peter?

3. What obligations would you, as a health care provider, have to keep Peter's condition strictly confidential?

■ Section Four: Inquiry and Exploration

PART 1: CRITICAL INQUIRY EXERCISES

1. Create a poster board illustrating the female and male reproductive systems. Indicate the reproductive disorders common to both sexes and those specific to one gender or the other.

2. Write a teaching plan addressing the learning needs of a 13-year-old who indicates a desire to become sexually active. What difference, if any, would the gender of the adolescent make in the plan?

PART 2: CRITICAL EXPLORATION EXERCISES

Arrange with your instructor to visit a health clinic that provides health care for adolescents who are sexually active. Note the health problems presented by the clients and identify the preventive measures provided by the professionals as they teach and counsel these clients.

CHAPTER 48

Nursing Care of the Child With an Endocrine or Metabolic Disorder

CHAPTER OVERVIEW

Chapter 48 reviews the care of the child with an endocrine or metabolic disorder. The chapter addresses the function of each hormone, the result of altered endocrine function, and a plan for nursing intervention. The case study helps the student understand the principles of assessing a child with an endocrine disorder.

LEARNING OBJECTIVES

After mastering the contents of this chapter, you should be able to:

1. Describe the structure and function of the different endocrine glands.

2. Assess a child with a disorder of endocrine function.

3. Formulate nursing diagnoses for a child with altered endocrine or metabolic function.

4. Develop appropriate outcomes for the child with endocrine or metabolic dysfunction.

5. Plan nursing care—for example, health teaching—for the child with altered endocrine or metabolic function.

6. Implement nursing care—for example, teaching insulin administration—for the child with an endocrine or metabolic disorder.

7. Evaluate outcomes to be certain that goals of nursing care were achieved.

8. Identify National Health Goals related to childhood endocrine or metabolic disorders that nurses could be instrumental in helping the nation achieve.

9. Identify areas related to care of children with endocrine or metabolic disorders that could benefit from additional nursing research or application of evidence-based practice.

10. Analyze ways that care of the child with altered endocrine or metabolic function can be family centered.

11. Synthesize knowledge of endocrine and metabolic dysfunctions and the nursing process to ensure quality maternal and child health nursing care.

KEY TERMS

carpal spasm	ketoacidosis
exophthalmos	latent tetany
glycosuria	manifest tetany
hormones	pedal spasm
hyperfunction	polydipsia
hyperglycemia	polyuria
hypofunction	sella turcica
hypoglycemia	Somogyi phenomenon
hypothalamus	

■ Section One:
Identification of Key Terms and Concepts

Match the terms in Part A with a definition or related statement from Part B. Place the letter corresponding to the answer in the space provided.

PART A

1. _____ Cushing's syndrome

2. _____ Latent tetany

3. _____ Polydipsia

4. _____ Galactosemia

5. _____ Hashimoto's disease

6. _____ Kussmaul breathing

7. _____ PKU

8. _____ Aldosterone

PART B

A. Excessive thirst

B. Acquired hypothyroidism

C. Secreted in response to renin-angiotensin

D. Overproduction of the adrenal hormone cortisol

E. Deep and rapid respirations

F. Neuromuscular irritability

G. Metabolic inherited disease

H. Disorder of carbohydrate metabolism

■ Section Two:
Short Answer and Completion Exercises

PART 1

Complete the following fill-in-the-blank exercises.

1. Type I (insulin-dependent) diabetes is characterized by almost no _____ secretion. The lack of insulin secretion contributes to a buildup of _____ in the bloodstream. If exogenous insulin is not administered, this person will develop _____ and _____.

2. Humulin-R insulin begins to work approximately _____ minutes after administration.

3. The peak action of Humulin R insulin is within _____ to _____ hours after administration.

4. Humulin N (NPH) insulin begins to work within _____ hours after administration.

5. Humulin N (NPH) insulin peaks within _____ to _____ hours after administration.

PART 2

Complete the following short answer questions.

1. What is the primary function of the endocrine system?

2. Each hormone of the endocrine system has a specific action. Complete the following chart by listing the hormones secreted from each of the glands and stating its action.

Gland	Hormones	Action
A. Pituitary		
B. Thyroid		
C. Adrenal		
D. Parathyroid		
E. Pancreas		

■ Section Three:
Critical Thinking for Application of Essential Concepts

PART 1

Circle the letter corresponding to the appropriate answer.

The nurse is counseling 10-year-old Shajuan and her parents in the hospital about the action of insulin and its effect upon the blood glucose levels before meals and at bedtime. The child has been instructed to take a split dose of regular and NPH insulin twice a day. The goal is to keep all glucose levels between 80 mg/dL and 150 mg/dL before meals. Shajuan has been instructed by the physician to change the insulin using pattern control.

1. Insulin causes the blood glucose to
   A. increase.
   B. decrease.
   C. neither increase nor decrease.
   D. increase, then decrease.

2. A pre-bedtime glucose level of 50 would be considered too low. The clinical symptoms would likely include which of the following?
   A. Thirst
   B. Flushing
   C. Dehydration
   D. Sweating

3. When a child begins to use an insulin pump, her parent must wake at 2 AM and test her for hypoglycemia. The reason the blood glucose may drop at this time may be too little
   A. food.
   B. exercise.
   C. fluid.
   D. sodium.

4. Shajuan has experienced Somogyi phenomenon. The following day Shajuan needs to consult with the physician and anticipate orders to
   A. increase the regular insulin.
   B. decrease the regular insulin.
   C. increase the intake of protein at supper.
   D. decrease the intake of protein at supper.

5. Shajuan is planning to play soccer at 3:00 in the afternoon. It would be best to
   A. take no insulin that morning.
   B. decrease regular insulin dosage in the morning.
   C. decrease NPH insulin dosage in the morning.
   D. increase the NPH insulin dosage in the morning.

6. Hypoglycemia may be caused by
   A. missing an insulin injection.
   B. missing a meal or a snack.
   C. too small an insulin dosage.
   D. too large a meal or snack.

PART 2: CASE STUDY

Ashley, age 5, is admitted to the children's hospital after her mom reports to the pediatrician that she has been urinating very frequently and has lost weight. Her mom also reports that she had several incidents of incontinence while playing on the playground. A careful history taken by the nurse revealed that Ashley's appetite had also increased. On admission to the hospital, laboratory studies were ordered. The results revealed a blood glucose level of 400 mg/dL.

1. The glucose tolerance test is ordered intravenously rather than orally. Why would the physician prefer this method?

2. What comfort measures should the nurse offer the child who is experiencing a fasting tolerance test?

3. What measures can be taken to lessen the discomfort for the diabetic child when frequent blood samples are needed?

▪ Section Four: Inquiry and Exploration

PART 1: CRITICAL INQUIRY EXERCISES

1. Create a blood glucose monitoring flow sheet. Be sure to include the date, blood glucose before each meal and bedtime, insulin dosage (both regular and NPH taken daily), and an explanation column where the patient can identify the reason for fluctuation in blood glucose.

2. Role play what it is like to check your blood glucose four times a day and record the amounts on your monitoring sheet. On the next day change the numbers to indicate hyperglycemia all day. Indicate what may have contributed to the problem.

PART 2: CRITICAL EXPLORATION EXERCISES

1. Attend a diabetes camp and offer to be a counselor in one of the cabins. Be sure to tell the camp director that diabetes is new to you and that you will need guidance.

2. Attend a meeting of the American Association of Diabetes Educators. Ask one of the certified diabetes educators about his or her job. How was certification obtained? Visit a diabetes education program that has been nationally recognized by the American Diabetes Association Advisory Council. Observe patient instructions and follow-up visits.

Nursing Care of the Child With a Neurologic Disorder

CHAPTER OVERVIEW

Chapter 49 discusses the care of the child with a neurologic disorder. The physiologic and psychological impact of common neurologic conditions on children at various stages of growth and development is discussed. The use of the nursing process to plan and provide care for the child with a neurologic disorder and his or her family is explored. The case study explores the nursing care of the child with a potentially life-threatening infection.

LEARNING OBJECTIVES

After mastering the contents of this chapter, you should be able to:

1. Describe common neurologic disorders in children.

2. Assess a child with a neurologic disorder.

3. Identify and address nursing diagnoses for the child with a neurologic disorder.

4. Identify National Health Goals for children who have neurologic disorders and elaborate on how nurses can help the identified population to achieve those goals.

5. Use critical thinking to analyze ways that care of the child with a neurologic disorder can be optimally family-centered.

6. Synthesize knowledge of neurologic disorders and the nursing process to achieve quality child health nursing care.

KEY TERMS

astereognosis
automatism
autonomic dysreflexia
autonomic nervous system (ANS)
central nervous system (CNS)
cerebrospinal fluid (CSF)
choreoathetosis
choreoid
decerebrate posturing
decorticate posturing
diplegia
doll's eye reflex

dyskinetic
dystonic
graphesthesia
hemiplegia
kinesthesia
neuron
paraplegia
peripheral nervous system (PNS)
pulse pressure
quadriplegia
status epilepticus
stereognosis

■ Section One:
Identification of Key Terms and Concepts

Match the terms in Part A with a definition or related statement from Part B. Place the letter corresponding to the answer in the space provided. (Letters may be used only once; some letters may not be used.)

PART A

1. _____ Electroencephalogram

2. _____ Graphesthesia

3. _____ Kinesthesia

4. _____ Ataxic

5. _____ Neurofibromatosis

6. _____ Diplegia

7. _____ Stereognosis

PART B

A. Awkward wide-base gait

B. Subcutaneous tumors along nerve pathways, with excessive skin pigmentation and possible optic or acoustic nerve degeneration

C. The ability to recognize a shape that has been traced on the skin

D. May require sedation for accurate measurement of the electrical patterns of the brain

E. The ability to distinguish movement

F. Child's arms are abducted and flexed on the chest with wrists flexed

G. Spastic cerebral palsy involvement affecting primarily the lower extremities

H. The ability to recognize an object by touch

■ Section Two:
Short Answer and Completion Exercises

Complete the following fill-in-the-blank exercises.

1. The nervous system consists of two separate systems, the _____ and the

    _____ nervous systems.

2. Tests for cerebellar function involve testing for normal _____ and

    _____.

3. Indicate if the following actions test sensory, motor, or cerebellar function.

    A. Asking a child to touch each finger on one hand with the thumb of that hand in rapid succession _____

    B. Asking a child to resist your action as you push down or up on his or her hands _____

    C. Touching the child's elbow with a vibrating tuning fork _____

4. The rate at which symptoms of intracranial pressure develop depends on the _____ and on whether the child's skull can _____ to accommodate the pressure.

5. Signs of _____ , in which a child is unsure of time and place, may be the first indication of increased intracranial pressure.

6. Cerebral perfusion pressure is calculated by subtracting the mean intracranial pressure from the mean _____ pressure.

7. The major cause of meningitis in newborns is the group B hemolytic _____ organism.

8. The treatment for infant botulism consists of _____ _____.

9. Convulsions associated with high fever are most common in _____ children between _____ months and _____ years of age.

10. Identify the seizure described below as psychomotor, absence, tonic-clonic, or simple partial.
   A. Generalized seizures with a prodromal, aural, tonic, and clonic stage
   _____

   B. Involves only one area of the brain; no altered level of consciousness
   _____

   C. May begin with a sudden change in posture, circumoral pallor, a 5-minute loss of consciousness without a postictal stage
   _____

   D. "Petit mal," generalized seizures involving a staring spell lasting for a few seconds _____

■ Section Three:
Critical Thinking for Application of Essential Concepts

PART 1

Circle the letter corresponding to the appropriate answer.

1. Melle, age 7, is admitted to your unit after an automobile accident. You would suspect increased intracranial pressure if your assessment revealed which of the following?
   A. Bradycardia rhythm
   B. Decreased pulse pressure
   C. Hypotensive blood pressure
   D. Tachypnea

2. A doll's eye reflex
   A. can be used to assess a comatose child neurologically.
   B. indicates increased intracranial pressure.

C. results when a child turns his or her eyes to the left as his or her head is turned to the left rapidly.

D. represents an abnormal neurologic finding.

3. Billy, age 2, has been diagnosed with cerebral palsy. The nurse should explain which of the following to Billy's parents?

A. Cerebral palsy involves a progressive nerve degeneration.

B. Contractures are unavoidable since ambulation is impossible.

C. The brain damage that occurred at birth can be repaired with surgery when the child is older.

D. Two children with cerebral palsy may exhibit totally different symptoms and abilities.

4. A child with Guillain-Barré syndrome will require which of the following nursing interventions?

A. Feeding the child orally to maintain the muscles of mastication

B. Explaining to parents that steroids will be effective in halting the paralysis

C. Immobilizing extremities to decrease stimulation of muscle spasm

D. Inserting a Foley catheter into the bladder to monitor urine output

5. To decrease the incidence of spinal cord injury in children and adolescents, the nurse should do which of the following?

A. Caution children and adolescents against diving into shallow water.

B. Encourage the intake of vitamins A and C to minimize spinal cord injury.

C. Instruct adolescents to ride motorcycles instead of driving cars.

D. Teach back exercises to children to strengthen their weak vertebrae.

6. A child with a cervical spinal injury should be watched very carefully for which of the following?

A. Diarrhea and hypoactive bowel sounds during the second recovery phase

B. Hyperreflexia of the bladder during the first recovery phase

C. Profuse diaphoresis during the second recovery phase

D. Respiratory distress during the first recovery phase

7. Which of the following are signs of autonomic dysreflexia?

A. Bradycardia and flushed face

B. Headache and hypertension

C. Hypertension and pallor

D. Pale skin and dizziness

8. Which of the following is true about the third phase of spinal cord recovery?

A. Autonomic dysreflexia is a common occurrence.

B. Spasticity of muscles and reflexes is noted.

C. Flaccid paralysis of the diaphragm and skeletal muscles is present.

D. Permanent limitation of motor and sensory function can be assessed.

9. Benje, age 7, is admitted to the emergency room with suspected spinal cord injury after an automobile accident. Which of the following nursing interventions would be appropriate?

    A. Move the child from the admission stretcher to a firm examining table on admission.

    B. Hyperextend the head if respiratory resuscitation is necessary.

    C. Remove any hard head coverings and replace with a support neck brace.

    D. Maintain spinal immobilization during neurologic assessments.

10. Nursing care of the spinal cord client may include which of the following interventions?

    A. Pushing carbonated beverages during the first phase of recovery to acidify urine

    B. Using Credé's maneuver to establish a defecation pattern

    C. Helping the child and family adjust to permanent mobility loss during the first recovery phase

    D. Supporting the child and family during the grieving process after the second recovery phase

PART 2

Determine if the following nursing interventions are appropriate or inappropriate. Indicate your answer by placing an "A" or an "I" in the space provided.

1. _____ Preparing a child with a suspected elevation of cerebral spinal fluid pressure for a lumbar puncture

2. _____ Pushing fluids after a lumbar puncture to reduce spinal headache

3. _____ Positioning a child flat in bed following myelography

4. _____ Monitoring a child undergoing an EEG for a possible seizure stimulated by use of the whirling disk

5. _____ Performing coughing exercises each hour with a child with increased intracranial pressure to keep chest clear

6. _____ Placing children with meningitis on droplet isolation for 24 hours after starting antibiotic therapy to prevent spread of the infection

7. _____ Teaching parents of children with meningitis to provide care and use proper isolation techniques

8. _____ Explaining to parents of a child with viral encephalitis that antibiotics will cure the infection

9. _____ Instructing the parent of a child with Reye's syndrome that the condition will run its course and requires no special treatment

10. _____ Teaching parents of children with seizures to place the child in a tub bath after a seizure episode to remove perspiration

PART 3: CASE STUDY

Mrs. Vereen has brought Shawn to the emergency room with an elevated temperature. Shawn is 4 years old and has had a cold for several days. Shawn's temperature on assessment was 104°F orally. He began to have a seizure during admission and was immediately taken to the treatment room. After some initial testing, he was diagnosed with *H. influenzae* meningitis.

1. How was the diagnosis confirmed?

2. Why should the nurse assess Shawn's skin for changes during assessments?

3. How is this disease treated? What is the impending complication if left untreated?

4. Should there be a concern for siblings and family members of the child with bacterial meningitis?

■ Section Four:
Inquiry and Exploration

PART 1: CRITICAL INQUIRY EXERCISES

1. Develop an abbreviated assessment for a soccer coach to assess an injured child with a mobility problem. Include advice the coach must give the persons who may want to assist him or her before professional help arrives.

2. Prepare a teaching plan stressing the importance of health care to prevent accidents; customize this plan to teach a parent group in a day-care setting. Include the National Health Goals as they relate to upper respiratory infections, the relationship of a disease and age frequency, and bike riding on streets.

PART 2: CRITICAL EXPLORATION EXERCISES

1. While on a pediatric clinical unit, perform a neurologic assessment on a client with no known neurologic conditions and on a client with a neurologic condition affecting neuromuscular or cerebral function. Note the differences in findings.

2. Observe the room of a client who has a history of seizures, or areas in which precautions should be taken, and note the seizure precautions taken for that client's safety.

Nursing Care of the Child With a Disorder of the Eyes or Ears

CHAPTER OVERVIEW

Chapter 50 discusses the eyes and ears as essential sensory organs. Disorders involving these organs in childhood may retard normal growth and development and, if untreated, may lead to long-term illness. This chapter addresses the structure of the eyes and ears, the physiology of vision and hearing, and common vision and hearing disorders, as well as the nurse's role in health promotion and management of vision and hearing disorders.

LEARNING OBJECTIVES

After mastering the contents of this chapter, you should be able to:

1. Describe the structure and function of the eyes and ears and disorders of these organs that affect children.

2. Assess the child who has a disorder of vision or hearing.

3. Formulate nursing diagnoses related to the child with a disorder of vision or hearing.

4. Establish appropriate outcomes for the child with a disorder of vision or hearing.

5. Plan nursing interventions for the child with a disorder of vision or hearing.

6. Implement nursing care to meet the specific needs of the child who has a disorder of the eyes or ears.

7. Evaluate outcomes for achievement and effectiveness of care.

8. Identify National Health Goals related to vision and hearing disorders of children that nurses could be instrumental in helping the nation achieve.

9. Identify areas related to care of children with vision or hearing disorders that could benefit from additional nursing research or application of evidence-based practice.

10. Use critical thinking to analyze ways that nursing care of children with a dysfunction of vision or hearing could be more family-centered.

11. Integrate knowledge of childhood disorders of the eyes or ears with the nursing process to achieve quality maternal and child health nursing care.

KEY TERMS

accommodation	light refraction
amblyopia	myopia
astigmatism	myringotomy
diplopia	nystagmus
enucleation	orthoptics
fovea centralis	ptosis
goniotomy	stereopsis
strabismus	tympanocentesis
hyperopia	

■ Section One: Identification of Key Terms and Concepts

PART 1

Match the terms in Part A with a definition or related statement from Part B. Place the letter corresponding to the answer in the space provided.

PART A

1. _____ Accommodation

2. _____ Chalazion

3. _____ Dacryostenosis

4. _____ Cerumen

5. _____ Ptosis

6. _____ Blepharitis marginalia

7. _____ Amblyopia

8. _____ Nystagmus

9. _____ Convergence

10. _____ Dacryocystitis

PART B

A. Turning both eyes medially

B. Infection of the eyelid margin

C. Inflammation of the nasolacrimal duct

D. Rapid, irregular eye movements

E. The inability to raise the upper eyelid normally

F. Interruption of the tear flow; blockage of the lacrimal drainage system

G. Serves to clean the external ear

H. Constriction of the pupil as it adjusts from focusing on a distant point to a near point

I. Low-grade granulation tissue tumor of the meibomian or tarsal gland on the eyelid

J. Reduced vision due to disuse of a structurally normal eye; sometimes referred to as "lazy eye"

PART 2

Indicate if the following statements are true or false by placing a "T" or "F" in the space provided.

1. _____ In the assessment of swimmer's ear, *Pseudomonas* and *Candida* are often found to be agents causing the infection.

2. _____ An internal ear canal altered by a fungal disease may appear brown or black.

3. _____ There is a higher incidence of otitis media in infants who are breast-fed than in those who are formula-fed.

4. _____ A myringotomy is a surgical procedure used to drain purulent fluids from an infected middle ear.

■ Section Two:
Short Answer and Completion Exercises

Complete the following fill-in-the-blank exercises.

1. _____ is the ability to locate an object in space relative to other objects.

2. Eye exercises are referred to as _____ .

3. _____ is a refractive error (farsightedness) in which vision is blurry at

   close range.

4. _____ is a congenital incomplete closure of the facial cleft.

■ Section Three:
Critical Thinking for Application of Essential Concepts

PART 1

Circle the letter corresponding to the appropriate answer.

1. The nurse should expect which of the following findings when assessing a child with acute otitis media?
   A. Excessive cerumen in the outer ear
   B. Recent respiratory tract infection
   C. Increased mobility on the pneumatic examination
   D. Copious amount of tenacious fluid

2. The primary cause of visual impairment in children is
   A. ocular trauma.
   B. exposure to elevated oxygen levels during infancy.
   C. congenital malformations.
   D. eye infection

3. To visualize the inner surface of a child's lower eyelid and most of the bottom globe, the nurse would
   A. pull the top eyelid outward and up.
   B. invert the top eyelid with a special apparatus.
   C. press on the lower lid with a finger tip.
   D. use a cotton tip to flip the lower lid.

4. If the ciliary body of the eye is involved with a penetration injury, sympathetic iritis may occur. This is described as
   A. a hemorrhagic paralysis.
   B. inflammation of the opposite eye.
   C. a global contusion.
   D. an infectious process of the globe.

5. Which of the following eye disorders in children can be definitely diagnosed by tonometry?
   A. Cataracts
   B. Diplopia
   C. Retinal detachment
   D. Glaucoma

6. A child is being surgically treated with a goniotomy procedure to provide an opening to the canal of Schlemm. Preoperatively, which of these drugs can be used to medically manage the client?
   A. Ampicillin
   B. Cephalosporin
   C. Diamox
   D. Maxidex

7. Which of the following impairment conditions is likely to occur as a sequela to untreated cataracts of infants?
   A. Amblyopia
   B. Dacryostenosis
   C. Astigmatism
   D. Keratitis

8. Surgery is stressful for all children, and emotional support should be included in the nurse's plan of care. Which of the following is a useful intervention to prepare the child before eye surgery?
   A. Showing the child a doll with patches over both eyes
   B. Restraining the child at the wrist bilaterally for 24 hours
   C. Avoiding discussion of the impending surgery
   D. Introducing the child to other children on the unit

PART 2: CASE STUDY

Ms. Jones's foster daughter Sally, age 6, was admitted to the hospital for surgery on the left eye. The presurgical diagnosis was a cataract of the left eye. The history and physical examination revealed that Sally's mother is a teenager and Sally has been in foster care since age 2. There was no medical history, and the laboratory and examination report stated that the lens of the left eye was opaque at the edges.

1. What would the nurse suspect as the etiology of the cataract?

2. In this condition would the retina appear red, black, or white?

3. Postoperatively, Sally complains of thirst; the postoperative orders read, "may have fluids when fully awake." When would the nurse allow Sally to have fluids, and why?

4. When teaching Ms. Jones postoperative care, what preventive measures would you want to address?

▪ Section Four:
Inquiry and Exploration

PART 1: CRITICAL INQUIRY EXERCISES

1. Prepare an interaction program for a school-age child who is hospitalized for a scheduled eye surgery. Focus on anticipatory guidance, before and after surgery. Incorporate measures to reduce anxiety, promote independence, and use parental participation.

2. Prepare a list of key points for parents to remember when interacting with their school-age child in the hospital environment.

PART 2: CRITICAL EXPLORATION EXERCISES

1. Make an appointment to visit the local support chapter for citizens who are deaf. Identify the support groups organized in cooperation with this agency. Note the teaching materials and classes made available to support the parents of the child with a hearing disability.

2. Visit a health clinic and participate in the hearing and vision screening for children entering school. Observe the steps taken when a child is found to have a vision or hearing problem.

CHAPTER 51

Nursing Care of the Child With a Musculoskeletal Disorder

CHAPTER OVERVIEW

Chapter 51 discusses the common musculoskeletal disorders experienced in childhood and the potential effects of these disorders on the child's growth and development. The use of the nursing process to plan and provide age-appropriate nursing care addressing the physiologic and psychological needs of the child with musculoskeletal disorders and of family members is explored.

LEARNING OBJECTIVES

After mastering the contents of this chapter, you should be able to:

1. Describe common musculoskeletal disorders in children.

2. Assess the child with a musculoskeletal disorder.

3. Use the nursing process to identify and address nursing diagnoses related to the child with a musculoskeletal disorder.

4. Identify National Health Goals related to musculoskeletal disorders and children that nurses can be instrumental in helping the nation achieve.

5. Identify areas related to care of the child with a musculoskeletal disorder that could benefit from additional nursing research.

6. Use critical thinking to analyze ways that care of the child immobilized by a cast or traction can be more family-centered.

7. Synthesize knowledge of musculoskeletal disorders with the nursing process to achieve quality child health nursing care.

KEY TERMS

apposition	metaphysis
arthroscopy	myopathy
cartilage	periosteum
diaphysis	petaling
distraction	remodeling
epiphyseal plate	reabsorption
epiphysis	sequestrum
fracture	smooth muscle
long bones	striated muscle
malleoli	traction

■ Section One: Identification of Key Terms and Concepts

Match the terms in Part A with a definition or related statement from Part B. Place the letter corresponding to the answer in the space provided. (Letters may be used only once; some letters will not be used.)

PART A

1. _____ Apposition
2. _____ Diaphysis
3. _____ Epiphyseal plate
4. _____ Genu varum
5. _____ Metaphysis
6. _____ Metatarsus adductus
7. _____ Myopathy
8. _____ Osteogenesis imperfecta
9. _____ Skeletal traction
10. _____ Striated muscle

PART B

A. Acquired or inherited disease in the muscular system
B. The muscle responsible for gastrointestinal peristalsis
C. The predominant muscle in the body; skeletal muscle
D. The cartilage segment at which increase in long bone length occurs
E. The thin area between the long bone shaft and the rounded end of the bone
F. The long central shaft of the long bone
G. Present when there is over an inch between the medial surfaces of the knees when standing with the malleoli of the ankles touching
H. The passing of a pin or wire through the skin into the end of the long bone
I. Placed on an infant to allow urine and feces to drain away from a cast
J. The amount of end-to-end contact of the bone fragments
K. Characterized by the formation of brittle bones
L. Turning in of the forefoot; can be corrected with stretching exercises

■ Section Two: Short Answer and Completion Exercises

PART 1

Complete the following fill-in-the-blank exercises.

1. A bone injury occurring at the _____ _____ of the long bone may result in irregular or abnormal bone length, and injury to the _____ or the bone may result in irregular bone width.

2. A broken femur in an adult will require 20 weeks to heal, whereas a toddler will heal in about _____ weeks.

3. Proper fitting of crutches requires a space of ___ to ____ inches between the axilla crutch pad and the child's axilla and elbow flexion of about ____ degrees.

4. Osgood-Schlatter disease is a _____ and _____ of the tibial tuberosity occurring in children who are athletic and at the _____ or _____ stage of development.

5. Apophysitis occurs most commonly in _____ who are growing rapidly. Pain produced by this condition can be treated by adding a _____ to the shoe heel to reduce tension on the heel cord.

6. To be classified as juvenile rheumatoid arthritis (JRA), symptoms must begin before ____ years of age and last longer than ____ months. The peak incidence occurs at two periods: between ___ and ___ years of age and ____ to ____ years of age.

7. During the periods of acute inflammation in JRA, joints should be _____ , but children may do _____ exercise.

PART 2

Complete the following short answer exercises.

1. Discuss why a child with a condition requiring a leg brace might have a nursing diagnosis of "Self-esteem disturbance."

2. What nursing measures could be taken to help a school-age child on complete bed rest with traction meet his developmental tasks?

3. Discuss two measures for managing itching underneath a cast and two measures that should not be used.

4. Discuss three exercises used to strengthen the foot arches of a child with flat feet.

5. Compare and contrast the causes of and the treatment for structural and functional scoliosis.

6. Describe the following types of braces and traction and the appropriate use of each:

Milwaukee brace

Halo traction

Bryant's traction

Buck's traction

Skeletal traction

■ Section Three:
Critical Thinking for Application of Essential Concepts

PART 1

Circle the letter corresponding to the appropriate answer.

1. Benji, age 11, has been diagnosed with osteomyelitis after a right leg injury 2 months ago. He and his parents were told he must be admitted to the hospital for treatment. The nurse should explain which of the following to Benji and his parents?

    A. Benji will need to ambulate immediately after surgery, although it may be uncomfortable.

    B. Blood will be drawn for culture to determine the specific medication for treatment of the infection.

    C. Infection control measures are necessary to prevent the spread of this condition to the entire family.

    D. The antibiotic therapy Benji will need must be administered IV and will be complete before discharge.

2. Legg-Calve-Perthes disease requires the implementation of which of the following nursing interventions?

    A. Discussing the use of surgery to make weight bearing possible and safe during 3 to 4 months of disease treatment

    B. Limiting ambulation to inside the room to decrease strain on weak leg muscles during the avascular necrosis disease stage

    C. Planning play activities that can be performed from the bed until after the reossification stage of the condition after 18 months

    D. Teaching weight-bearing exercises to be performed every 4 hours during the revascularization stage of the disease

3. Amy, 3 years old, has been diagnosed with osteogenesis imperfecta. When planning her care, the nurse should consider which of the following?

    A. Active range-of-motion and weight lifting exercises will be necessary to strengthen weak long bone shafts.

    B. Amy's parents should be encouraged to facilitate her development by not restricting her activities.

    C. Genetic counseling will be appropriate if Amy's condition is congenital or late-occurring.

    D. The treatment for this condition requires lifelong oral intake of calcium supplements.

4. When teaching Sheila, 13 years old, to walk with crutches, the nurse should instruct her to

    A. move one crutch forward at a time when using a three-point swing-through gait.

    B. rest the crutch pad on the upper arm to bear her weight on the axilla crutch pad.

    C. carry books and other items in a backpack to keep her hands free.

    D. use a two-point gait when no weight bearing is allowed.

5. Marla, age 12, has a cast on her left leg. During a follow-up phone call, Marla states she is experiencing occasional numbness in her left foot and the foot feels cool. The nurse should respond in which of the following ways?

   A. Explain to Marla that she needs to wiggle her toes frequently to prevent the return of the numbness and coolness.

   B. Inform Marla and her mother of the need to elevate the extremity to promote good circulation.

   C. Instruct Marla and her mother to return to the doctor for possible removal of the cast.

   D. Teach Marla isometric exercises to use when numbness and coolness occur.

6. The nurse would determine that the plan of care for a child with juvenile rheumatoid arthritis (JRA) had been effective if which of the following findings was noted?

   A. The parents state the need to avoid aspirin administration to prevent Reye's syndrome.

   B. Meals are offered after periods of rest and administration of pain medication and are 80% eaten.

   C. Splints are applied during the day and removed at night by parents to promote sleep.

   D. Ice baths are applied to the affected joints by parents twice daily.

7. A care plan for a girl suspected of having myasthenia gravis may include which of the following?

   A. Administering cholinergic drugs to suppress the hyperactivity actions of acetylcholine

   B. Inquiring if the child has had difficulty in school recently due to difficulty reading or seeing the board

   C. Reassuring the adolescent female that myasthenia gravis will not affect her childbearing potential

   D. Scheduling medications after mealtime to decrease gastrointestinal symptoms, choking, and possible aspiration

8. Congenital muscular dystrophy differs from Duchenne's disease and facioscapulohumeral muscular dystrophy in which of the following ways?

   A. Congenital muscular dystrophy results in degeneration of muscle fibers.

   B. Congenital muscular dystrophy can result in problems with parental bonding.

   C. In facioscapulohumeral muscular dystrophy, the predominant symptom is facial weakness.

   D. Victims of Duchenne's disease and their families should have genetic counseling.

PART 2

Determine if the following nursing interventions are appropriate or inappropriate for the child undergoing spinal instrumentation for treatment of scoliosis. Indicate your answer by placing an "A" or an "I" in the space provided.

1. _____ Maintain the head of the bed at a 45-degree elevation.

2. _____ Logroll the child to a side-lying position every 2 hours unless Luque/segmented rods are used.

3. _____ Monitor the neurologic and vascular function of the extremities every hour for the first 24 hours.

4. _____ Explain the need to keep the child NPO until bowel sounds are audible.

5. _____ Instruct the parents not to touch the child during the early postoperative period.

6. _____ Reassure the child that although the rods usually remain in place permanently, they are not obvious to others.

7. _____ Instruct the child that good posture is mandatory and to bend at the knees to remove objects from the floor.

8. _____ Reassure the child that moderate movement is safe after final cast removal following rod insertion.

9. _____ Explain to parents that even severe scoliosis can be completely corrected with surgery.

10. _____ Inform female clients with scoliosis that child-bearing is contraindicated.

PART 3: CASE STUDY

Evelyn Demark, 10 years old, has osteogenesis imperfecta and is admitted to your unit with a fracture of the right forearm due to an injury in gymnastics class.

1. What would you need to discuss during your teaching session with Evelyn and her parents related to activity choices?

2. How would Evelyn's plan of care differ if she did not have osteogenesis imperfecta?

■ Section Four: Inquiry and Exploration

PART 1: CRITICAL INQUIRY EXERCISES

1. Write a care plan for a school-age child hospitalized with bilateral leg traction after an accident. Include age-appropriate activities.

2. What safety and development issues would you include in a teaching plan for a 7-month-old with a broken femur due to a fall down the stairs at home?

PART 2: CRITICAL EXPLORATION EXERCISES

Walk through your home and the home of a friend. Note any circumstances that could represent a danger to a child.

CHAPTER 52

Nursing Care of the Child With a Traumatic Injury

CHAPTER OVERVIEW

Accidents are a major cause of childhood morbidity and mortality, and prevention is a goal that nurses and other health care providers always strive for. However, not all accidents can be prevented. Chapter 51 describes the principles of nursing care for the child with a traumatic injury. The uses of the nursing process to assess, plan, and provide appropriate nursing care and to address the physiologic and psychological needs of the child and family involved with traumatic injury are discussed.

LEARNING OBJECTIVES

After mastering the contents of this chapter, you should be able to:

1. Describe the causes and consequences of common accidents and injuries in childhood, as well as measures to prevent them.

2. Assess a child injured from an accident such as poisoning or burning.

3. Use the nursing process to identify and address nursing diagnoses related to the injured child.

4. Identify National Health Goals related to children and trauma that nurses can be instrumental in helping the nation achieve.

5. Use critical thinking to analyze ways that accidents and injuries can be prevented in childhood.

6. Synthesize knowledge of injuries in childhood with the nursing process to achieve quality child health nursing care.

KEY TERMS

allografting
autografting
contrecoup injury
debridement
drowning
escharotomy
heterografts

homografting
near-drowning
otorrhea
plumbism
rhinorrhea
stupor

■ Section One:
Identification of Key Terms and Concepts

Match the terms in Part A with a definition or related statement from Part B. Place the letter corresponding to the answer in the space provided. (Letters may be used only once; some letters may not be used.)

PART A

1. _____ Allografting

2. _____ Chelating agents

3. _____ Contrecoup injury

4. _____ Contusion

5. _____ Escharotomy

6. _____ Heterografting

7. _____ Leptomeningeal cyst

8. _____ Plumbism

9. _____ Rhinorrhea

10. _____ Stupor

PART B

A. Cutting into the tough leathery scab over a burned area to release a tight band around an extremity

B. Placing of skin from cadavers or a donor on a cleaned burn site

C. A tearing or laceration of brain tissue, with symptoms specific to the brain area affected

D. Grogginess from which an individual can be roused

E. Lead poisoning; usually occurs in toddlers and preschool children

F. Clear fluid draining from the nose; if it is cerebrospinal fluid it will be positive for glucose

G. A concussion on the side of the brain opposite that which was struck; occurs as the brain recoils from the force of the blow

H. Skin from a nonhuman source, such as porcine (pig), used to promote skin growth after a burn

I. Skin taken from an unburned area of a burn victim's body and placed on a prepared burned area to facilitate healing

J. Substances that act to remove lead from soft tissue and bone and eliminate it in the urine

K. Results from projection of the arachnoid membrane into the fracture site; may cause symptoms of increased intracranial pressure

■ Section Two:
Short Answer and Completion Exercises

PART 1

Complete the following fill-in-the-blank exercises.

1. The extent of a child's injury depends on _____ , _____ , and _____ .

2. The Glasgow Coma Scale includes assessment of _____ _____ , responses to speech and pain, and _____ and _____ responses.

3. _____ _____-degree burns are not extremely painful.

4. Equipment used to care for a severely burned child must be _____ to prevent wound infection.

5. Second- or third-degree burns may be cared for by _____ treatment, which involves leaving the burned area exposed to air.

6. Nurses can help the nation meet health goals concerned with trauma by being _____ care providers who provide counseling on _____ _____ to parents and _____ .

PART 2

Complete the following short answer exercises.

1. Discuss the appropriate method for discharge teaching of parents of injured children discharged from the emergency room.

2. Explain why the "rule of nines" cannot be used to determine the extent of burns on infants and children.

3. Discuss the reason burn injuries to the face and throat can be more hazardous than other burn injuries.

4. Describe the infection control measures used for burn victims.

5. Describing the appropriate emergency treatment for the indicated burn injuries:

First-degree

Second- and third-degree

Electrical burn

Facial or neck burns

■ Section Three:
Critical Thinking for Application of Essential Concepts

PART 1

Circle the letter corresponding to the appropriate answer.

1. Which of the following would be a serious danger sign if noted in a child after head trauma?
   A. Complaint of headache along the area of trauma
   B. Blood pressure moving from 120/80 to 130/50
   C. Memory deficit with inability to recall time or date
   D. Pupils equal and briskly reactive to light

2. Care of the child in a coma would include
   A. Encouraging parents to be positive since coma is often short term in children.
   B. Performing passive range-of-motion exercises to maintain muscle tone.
   C. Feeding the child with a spoon and fork to stimulate memories of normal activity.
   D. Maintaining the child in a flat, supine position to simulate normal sleeping position.

3. Jan, age 13, is admitted with third-degree burns over 25% of her body. Which of the following is an immediate concern in Jan's plan of care?

   A. Liberal medication to control Jan's severe pain

   B. Arranging age-appropriate diversional activities

   C. Preventing hypovolemia and circulatory collapse

   D. Increasing oral intake of proteins to build tissue

4. A realistic outcome criterion for the parents of a child who is the victim of traumatic injury would be for the parents to

   A. admit responsibility for the child's trauma.

   B. allow the child to perform household chores without supervision to strengthen self-esteem.

   C. prevent all future accidental childhood injury.

   D. state measures they can take to prevent common accidents from occurring.

PART 2

Determine if the nursing intervention described for the specified trauma is appropriate or inappropriate. Indicate your answer by placing the letter "A" or "I" in the space provided.

1. _____ Subdural hematoma: Monitor for seizures, vomiting, or hyperirritability for up to 20 days after the trauma.

2. _____ Concussion: Instruct parents not to allow the child to sleep for 24 hours after the trauma.

3. _____ Acetaminophen poisoning: Administer syrup of ipecac followed by acetylcysteine/Mucomyst in a carbonated drink.

4. _____ Caustic poisoning: Administer syrup of ipecac followed by cold water or milk.

5. _____ Hydrocarbon ingestion: Monitor the child for respiratory irritation.

6. _____ Iron poisoning: Monitor for initial nausea, diarrhea, and abdominal pain followed by melena and hematemesis and shock 12 hours later.

7. _____ Lead poisoning: Instruct parents to repaint the home before the child is discharged.

8. _____ Plant poisoning: Reassure parents that this is not serious and requires no treatment.

9. _____ Recreational drug poisoning: Attempt to determine if the ingestion was a suicide attempt if the child is over 7 years of age.

10. _____ Foreign body obstruction: Irrigate the child's ear canal with saline to remove a peanut.

11. _____ Frostbite: Place the affected body part in hot water to restore circulation immediately.

12. _____ Snake bite: Apply a cold compress to the site immediately and keep the site in a dependent position to slow venom spread; monitor for bruising and bleeding.

13. _____ Facial burn: Monitor for stridor or other signs of respiratory tract obstruction.

14. _____ Third-degree burn over 10% of the body: Decrease fluid intake to aid kidneys in filtration of waste and concentration of urine.

15. _____ Any traumatic injury: Restrict parental involvement in care of the child to decrease demands on parents.

PART 3: CASE STUDY

Mr. and Mrs. Chin come to your emergency room with their 3-year-old son, Jay. Jay is an active child who has broken his arm and sprained a wrist climbing on furniture. Jay likes to ride his tricycle around the house and yard and once nearly drank a liquid cleaner that was not placed out of reach in the kitchen. Jay's arm is placed in a cast.

1. What psychological supports would you need to provide for Jay and his parents to help them cope with the current injury and plan for Jay's continued development?

2. What safety issues would you need to address with the Chin family, and what further assessments would you make?

3. What age-appropriate activities would you suggest to the Chin family to facilitate Jay's development?

■ Section Four: Inquiry and Exploration

PART 1: CRITICAL INQUIRY EXERCISES

1. What safety suggestions could you give to a couple who have open fireplaces and space heaters in their home and three active children ages 18 months, 3 years, and 5 years?

2. Prepare a plan of care addressing outdoor summer activities and dress for parents of a child who lives on a ranch in the Southwest.

PART 2: CRITICAL EXPLORATION EXERCISES

1. Visit a burn center and observe the care measures taken for clients at various ages and with various types and degrees of burns.

2. Locate the names and phone numbers of the emergency medical system and the poison control center in your neighborhood.

CHAPTER 53

Nursing Care of the Child With Cancer

CHAPTER OVERVIEW

The diagnosis of cancer in a child can be devastating to a family. However, the prognosis for children with cancer is continually improving. Chapter 53 provides an overview of the special care needs of the child with cancer. The physical and psychological effects of various types of childhood cancers are discussed. The use of the nursing process to plan and provide care for the child and the family coping with cancer is explored.

LEARNING OBJECTIVES

After mastering the contents of this chapter, you should be able to:

1. Define terms related to tumor growth such as neoplasm, benign, malignant, sarcoma, and carcinoma, and describe normal cell growth and theories that explain how cells are altered to become neoplastic in children.

2. Assess the child with a neoplastic process such as a rhabdomyosarcoma, neuroblastoma, Wilms' tumor, or leukemia.

3. Use the nursing process to identify and address nursing diagnoses related to the child with a malignancy.

4. Identify National Health Goals related to children and cancer that nurses can be instrumental in helping the nation achieve.

5. Use critical thinking to analyze ways that nursing care for the child with a neoplasm can be more family-centered.

6. Synthesize knowledge of abnormal cell growth in children with the nursing process to achieve quality child health nursing care.

KEY TERMS

biopsy
chemotherapeutic agent
Ewing's sarcoma
leukemia
lymphoma
metastasis
neoplasm

neuroblastoma
oncogenic virus
oncogenic virusosteogenic sarcoma
rhabdomyosarcoma
sarcoma
tumor staging

■ Section One:
Identification of Key Terms and Concepts

Match the terms in Part A with a definition or related statement from Part B. Place the letter corresponding to the answer in the space provided.

PART A

1. _____ Alopecia

2. _____ Allogeneic

3. _____ Ependymoma

4. _____ Glioma

5. _____ Neoplasm

6. _____ Neuroblastoma

7. _____ Oncogenic

8. _____ Osteogenic sarcoma

9. _____ Rhabdomyosarcoma

10. _____ Staging

PART B

A. A term commonly used for a new abnormal growth that does not respond to growth control mechanisms

B. Cancer-causing agent

C. Hair loss; occurs secondary to almost all chemotherapeutic cancer drugs

D. A transplant between a histocompatible person and a child with cancer

E. Designating the extent of a malignant process

F. A tumor arising from the floor of the fourth ventricle of the brain

G. A tumor of the support tissue of the brain

H. A tumor of striated muscle

I. A tumor arising from the cells of the sympathetic nervous system

J. A malignant tumor of long bone involving rapidly growing bone tissue

■ Section Two:
Short Answer and Completion Exercises

PART 1

Complete the following fill-in-the-blank exercises.

1. Carcinogens can be _____ , _____ , or _____ agents.

2. Because cells lining the stomach are fast-growing, _____ and _____ are common side effects of chemotherapy.

3. Chemotherapy for acute lymphatic leukemia is given first in a _____ phase, next in a _____ phase, and finally in a _____ phase.

4. Early symptoms in children with leukemia are _____ , _____ , and _____ .

5. Hodgkin's disease is confirmed by _____ _____ and _____ of the _____ .

6. An adolescent with osteosarcoma who must undergo leg amputation might achieve the goal of realizing the amputation is _____ to save _____ _____ .

7. _____ _____ is a malignant tumor occurring most often in the bone marrow of the midshaft of long bones.

8. _____ is a rare malignant tumor of the eye.

9. _____ may be needed as treatment for retinoblastoma if the tumor is large.

10. Neuroblastomas may cause loss of motor function due to _____ on the spinal nerves or _____ into the intervertebral foramina.

PART 2

Complete the following short answer exercises.

1. Describe five of the common categories of chemotherapeutic cancer agents.

2. Discuss factors that may contribute to decreased nutritional status in a child with cancer.

3. Discuss the treatment of Hodgkin's disease for children at stage I or II at the time of diagnosis, stage III at the time of diagnosis, and stage IV at the time of diagnosis.

■ Section Three:
Critical Thinking for Application of Essential Concepts

PART 1

Circle the letter corresponding to the appropriate answer.

1. Mrs. Peters states she's glad her son Tim's cancer was caught early and now he is safe from cancer in later life. The nurse should respond with which of the following principles in mind?

   A. Cancer is less likely to strike Tim again.

   B. Childhood cancer usually instills an immunity to cancer.

   C. Children surviving one cancer have a greater risk for a second cancer.

   D. Cancer onset is unpredictable and carries no pattern of recurrence.

2. Children with cancer would be most vulnerable for skeletal side effects from radiation therapy at which of the following ages?

   A. 2 years

   B. 4 years

   C. 6 years

   D. 12 years

3. Which of the following is true about radiation therapy?

   A. The skin areas at which the radiotherapy is directed should be washed daily with soap and water.

   B. Creams and lotions should not be applied to the radiation site until a radiation series is complete.

   C. Sedatives and analgesics should be withheld during radiotherapy.

   D. Radiation may result in excessive salivary gland function.

4. Which of the following nursing interventions is most important when caring for a child receiving vincristine?

   A. Administering salicylates to relieve nerve pain

   B. Encouraging intake of high-fiber foods

   C. Monitoring for frequent diarrheal stools

   D. Planning age-appropriate coloring or drawing activities

5. The decreased platelet production from leukemia's effect on a child's bone marrow would result in which of the following symptoms?

   A. Flushed skin

   B. Epistaxis

   C. Hyperthermia

   D. Tachycardia

6. Children who have a brain tumor will have which of the following symptoms?
   A. Abdominal pain
   B. Diarrhea
   C. Hypotension
   D. Vomiting

7. Which of the following interventions may be needed for the parents of a child diagnosed with a brain tumor?
   A. Allowing the parents to delay treatment for weeks if needed until the denial stage resolves
   B. Explaining that removal of a small peripheral tumor is a minor surgical procedure
   C. Reinforcing preoperative explanations about the nature of the child's diagnosis after surgery is over
   D. Reassuring parents that radiation and chemotherapy can cure brain tumors and prevent metastasis

8. A child with a neuroblastoma
   A. frequently experiences bone metastasis to the bone marrow.
   B. has a good chance of survival if diagnosed with stage I or II disease.
   C. often has frequent intense headaches and diplopia.
   D. will most likely be school-age or adolescent.

PART 2

Determine if the following nursing interventions are appropriate or inappropriate. Indicate your answer by placing an "A" or an "I" in the space provided.

1. _____ Encouraging children receiving chemotherapy to take clear fluids, even if they are nauseated, to prevent uric acid buildup in the kidney

2. _____ Using ice packs to the scalp of children with leukemia to decrease alopecia

3. _____ Placing a child receiving immunosuppressive drugs on wound and skin isolation to minimize spread of infection

4. _____ Placing a warm compress on a site of infiltration of a chemotherapeutic agent

5. _____ Administering live virus vaccines to immunosuppressed children to achieve maximum protection against infection

6. _____ Pushing fluids with children receiving chemotherapy to reduce loss of kidney function

7. _____ Monitoring a child receiving chemotherapy for leukemia for nuchal rigidity, headache, irritability, and vomiting

8. _____ Encouraging normal activity and regular school for children in the maintenance phase of leukemia therapy

9. _____ Administering pneumococcal vaccine to children with Hodgkin's disease who have had a splenectomy

10. _____ Reassuring the parents of a child having surgery for removal of a brain tumor that the child will be awake and oriented after surgery

PART 3: CASE STUDY

Mr. and Mrs. Morrell have been advised that Joseph has a brain tumor. He was admitted 2 days ago for preoperative lab work. Today is the day of the surgery, and you are assigned as Joseph's operating room nurse. When reading the surgical checklist, you found that Joseph had not received an enema or any methods to evacuate the bowel.

1. What would be your response after learning of this situation?

2. Provide a rationale for each of these postoperative orders for Joseph: NPO, keep HOB elevated 45 degrees, position on side, administer eye drops q4h, neuro checks q2h, change dressing when wet, monitor vital signs, D5 1/4 NS to KVO.

■ Section Four: Inquiry and Exploration

PART 1: CRITICAL INQUIRY EXERCISES

1. Prepare a teaching plan for a child with a diagnosis of leukemia or her parents.

2. Develop a tool to contrast the presenting symptoms that may be seen on an assessment for a child presenting with leukemia. The tool should help you determine the type of malignancy based on the clinical picture.

PART 2: CRITICAL EXPLORATION EXERCISES

Visit a pediatric cancer ward. Note the varied types of childhood cancer and the types of medical and nursing treatments being provided.

The Nursing Role in Restoring and Maintaining the Health of Children and Families With Mental Health Disorders

CHAPTER 54

Nursing Care of the Child With a Cognitive or Mental Health Disorder

CHAPTER OVERVIEW

Children who are cognitively impaired have the same fundamental needs as other children. The nurse has a responsibility to provide the families of these children with skills to observe, solve problems, make decisions, and prevent illness. This chapter presents common illnesses, identifies behaviors, and explores methods of helping the family manage.

LEARNING OBJECTIVES

After mastering the contents of this chapter, you should be able to:

1. Describe common cognitive and mental health disorders in children.

2. Assess a child for a cognitive or mental health disorder.

3. Formulate nursing diagnoses related to the cognitive or mental health disorders of childhood.

4. Establish appropriate outcomes for the child with a cognitive or mental health disorder.

5. Plan nursing care for the child with a cognitive or mental health disorder.

6. Implement nursing care for the child with a cognitive or mental health disorder.

7. Evaluate outcomes for achievement and effectiveness of care.

8. Identify National Health Goals related to cognitive or mental health disorders that nurses can be instrumental in helping the nation achieve.

9. Identify areas related to cognitive or mental health that could benefit from additional nursing research or application of evidence-based practice.

10. Analyze ways that care of the child with a cognitive or mental health disorder can be more family-centered.

11. Integrate knowledge of childhood cognitive and mental health disorders and nursing process to achieve quality maternal and child health nursing care.

KEY TERMS

anhedonia

binge eating

catatonia

choreiform movements

complex vocal tics

coprolalia

dyslexia

echolalia

expressed emotion

flat affect

graphesthesia

hyperactivity

labile mood

motor tics

palilalia

purging

school phobia

stereognosis

vocal tics

■ Section One: Identification of Key Terms and Concepts

PART 1

Match the terms in Part A with a definition or related statement from Part B. Place the letter corresponding to the answer in the space provided.

PART A

1. _____ Encopresis

2. _____ Motor tics

3. _____ Catatonia

4. _____ Dyslexia

5. _____ Tourette's disease

PART B

A. Muscle movements such as rapid repetitive eye blinking or facial twitching

B. Inherited syndrome of facial and complex vocal tics

C. Passing feces in culturally unacceptable places

D. A learning disorder involving reading disability

E. Behavior manifestation seen in children with schizophrenia, characterized by withdrawal and stuporous depression

PART 2

Indicate if the following statements are true or false by placing "T" or "F" in the space provided.

1. _____ Assessment of retardation can be conclusively measured by an appropriate IQ test, preferably the Stanford Binet.

2. _____ A severely retarded child may need to be institutionalized, since obtaining baby-sitters is difficult and these children must have constant supervision.

3. _____ Separation anxiety in an 18-month-old child is a sign of developmental delay.

4. _____ Children who experience "normal" sadness often report being unable to remember the last time they were happy.

■ Section Two:
Short Answer and Completion Exercises

Complete the following short answer questions.

1. List the criteria for mental retardation as described by DSM-IV-TR.

2. Define labile mood.

3. Describe graphesthesia, stereognosis, and choreiform.

4. State the term that describes the eating of nonfood substances such as dirt, clay, and crayons.

■ Section Three:
Critical Thinking for Application of Essential Concepts

PART 1

Circle the letter corresponding to the appropriate answer.

1. All of the following characteristics are descriptive of the child with attention deficit hyperactivity disorder (ADHD) except

    A. hypoactivity.

    B. attentiveness

    C. impulsiveness.

    D. conscientiousness.

2. When providing anticipatory guidance to parents of a hyperactive child, the nurse would encourage them to

   A. assign chores appropriate to the child's age.

   B. be flexible and lenient regarding limits.

   C. give instructions to this child in the group setting with the other siblings.

   D. delay punishing the child to allow the child time to think about mistakes.

3. Baby girl Franshon, 12 months old, is admitted to the hospital for electrolyte imbalance and R/O abdominal obstruction. After careful assessment the physician describes Baby Franshon as regurgitating her food after ingestion and then reswallowing it. Research postulates that this is a form of self-stimulation by the infant. This disorder is termed

   A. encopresis.

   B. rumination.

   C. anhedonia.

   D. bulimia.

4. Felicia is 15 years old and is admitted to the hospital with anorexia nervosa. She is a model and often spoken of as an overachiever. As the nurse interviews Felicia and her family, she may discover other characteristics such as

   A. early development of secondary sex characteristics.

   B. permissive parenting.

   C. amenorrhea.

   D. hyperglycemia.

5. Which of the following is commonly seen in children with anorexia nervosa?

   A. Morbid obesity

   B. Ingesting copious amounts of water

   C. Body mass index above 85% of expected

   D. Binge eating and purging

6. A child with an IQ of 44 would be categorized as having which type of mental retardation?

   A. Mild

   B. Moderate

   C. Severe

   D. Profound

PART 2: CASE STUDY

Stephen is 2½ years old; his mother brings him to the health clinic with an ear infection. The history and physical exam reveal that Stephen's behavior is quite different from that of the other siblings. The mother reports that he hates to be held, only utters sounds when trying to talk, gets upset easily, and screams constantly. You notice that Stephen has excoriated lesions on his thumbs.

1. Based on the information, what would be a probable diagnosis for Stephen?

2. What type of temperament is usually seen with these children?

3. How can the nurse assist the parents in bonding with Stephen and providing developmental support?

■ Section Four:
Inquiry and Exploration

PART 1: CRITICAL INQUIRY EXERCISES

1. Arrange with your instructor to invite to your classroom the mother of an 8-year-old or older child with a cognitive or mental health disorder. Ask her to explain how she prepares the child for health visits and what she does in the household to protect the child from injury.

2. Develop an assessment tool to be used in a clinical setting to help the health care professional recognize the signs and symptoms of teenage depression.

PART 2: CRITICAL EXPLORATION EXERCISES

Attend a school that has an academic or vocational curriculum for the retarded student. Research the activities in the curriculum that will help the student become a functional member of his or her community and society.

CHAPTER 55

Nursing Care of the Family in Crisis: Abuse and Violence in the Family

CHAPTER OVERVIEW

Child and domestic abuse is a national problem with serious consequences for children. Chapter 55 describes the physiologic and psychological effects of child and domestic abuse. The use of the nursing process to identify, plan, and provide appropriate nursing care to help victims and their family members or significant others cope with the trauma of child and domestic abuse is discussed.

LEARNING OBJECTIVES

After mastering the contents of this chapter, you should be able to:

1. Discuss the types of abuse seen in families and the theories explaining them.

2. Assess a physically or emotionally abused family.

3. Use the nursing process to identify and address nursing diagnoses related to the abused family.

4. Identify National Health Goals related to child abuse that nurses can be instrumental in helping the nation achieve.

5. Identify areas related to care of the abused child that could benefit from additional nursing research.

6. Use critical thinking to analyze ways that nurses can be instrumental in preventing child abuse.

7. Synthesize knowledge of family abuse with the nursing process to achieve quality child health nursing care.

KEY TERMS

abuse	Munchausen syndrome by proxy
disorganization phase	pedophile
failure to thrive	permissive reporters
incest	rape trauma syndrome
intimate partner abuse	reorganization syndrome
learned helplessness	shaken baby syndrome
mandatory reporters	silent rape syndrome
molestation	

■ Section One:
Identification of Key Terms and Concepts

Match the terms in Part A with a definition or related statement from Part B. Place the letter corresponding to the answer in the space provided. (Use each letter once; some letters may not be used.)

PART A

1. _____ Abuse

2. _____ Disorganization phase

3. _____ Battered child syndrome

4. _____ Mandatory reporters

5. _____ Molestation

6. _____ Munchausen syndrome by proxy

7. _____ Pedophile

8. _____ Psychological infantilism

9. _____ Shaken baby syndrome

PART B

A. Severe abuse and victims of disability

B. Learned helplessness; being obedient and cooperative in an effort to reduce the violence

C. Parents who repeatedly bring a child to a health care facility reporting symptoms of illness when, in fact, the child is well

D. Willful injury of one person by another

E. The first stage of rape trauma syndrome; lasts about 3 days

F. The second stage of rape trauma syndrome; may last months or years

G. People who must notify the authorities of suspected abuse; nurses fall into this category

H. Sexual involvement between an adult and child, such as oral-genital contact or viewing genitals

I. An adult who seeks out children for sexual gratification

J. Whiplash injury to the neck, edema to the brain stem, retinal hemorrhages, and potential respiratory arrest

K. A disturbance in the parent-child relationship that might contribute to failure to thrive

■ Section Two: Short Answer and Completion Exercises

PART 1

Complete the following fill-in-the-blank exercises.

1. _____ is often the first person to identify the symptoms of possible child abuse.

2. The triad of circumstances that generally combine to result in child abuse are a _____ _____ , a child seen as _____ in the parent's eyes, and a _____ _____ or circumstance.

3. Excessive use of _____ by the abusive person is strongly associated with abuse.

4. When questioned about an injury, an abused child will usually _____ the parent's story.

PART 2

Complete the following short answer exercises.

1. Discuss why children in an abusive family situation might have other undiagnosed medical problems.

2. Discuss one major reason why victims of child abuse might grow to be abusers themselves.

3. Why should a nurse examine his or her personal feelings related to the abuser and the victim in a domestic abuse situation?

4. Discuss one method of differentiating between organic and nonorganic failure to thrive.

5. List symptoms of infants demonstrating failure to thrive relative to physical and social development.

■ Section Three:
Critical Thinking for Application of Essential Concepts

PART 1

Circle the letter corresponding to the appropriate answer.

1. Because abuse involves and affects all the members of a family, the nurse should have which of the following as part of the care plan goals?

   A. Disrupting the dysfunctional family

   B. Improving overall family functioning

   C. Punishing the abusive family member

   D. Removing the abuse victim from the family

2. When planning a strategy to address child and domestic abuse, the nurse should do which of the following?

   A. Lecture parents suspected of child abuse on the evils of violence.

   B. Report suspected child abuse whenever a child with bruises is admitted.

   C. Stop parental visitation immediately if child abuse is suspected.

   D. Work with pregnant teen groups to teach parenting skills.

3. At his first physical, Bob, 14 years old, stated that the multiple long whip-like scars on his back occurred as a result of falling backward against a rough bedroom floor when he was playing with a friend. The nurse should respond in which of the following ways?

   A. Ask additional questions regarding the cause of the injury and any other injuries noted.

   B. Discuss with Bob the fact that his clumsiness is probably a part of his adolescence and that he will outgrow it.

   C. Instruct Bob in the importance of exercise and good nutrition to avoid easy bruising.

   D. Tell Bob you do not believe him and you want to know if his parents caused his injuries.

4. Sheila, 11 years old, is admitted with vaginal bleeding. The nurse notices that Sheila and her mother are very nervous but state that they are "sure it's just menstrual blood." The nurse should initially do which of the following?

   A. Accept the fact that Sheila is probably beginning menses; don't jump to conclusions.

   B. Explain to Sheila and her mother that menstrual bleeding does not occur at this early age.

   C. Insist that Sheila's mother tell if someone is abusing Sheila.

   D. Gently examine Sheila for torn perineal tissue or lacerations.

5. Which of the following would place a parent at high risk for being a child abuser?

   A. Being poor and a member of a minority group

   B. Choosing to have a baby without being married

   C. Having less than a high school education

   D. Severe disappointment with the sex of a new baby

6. Daryl, age 7, states he can't tell about his father's beating him because the beating will get worse. The nurse should remember which of the following when replying to Daryl?

   A. Daryl might be angry with his parents and making up this story.

   B. Daryl's mother can protect him from the father if necessary.

   C. Most institutions can hold a child for 72 hours for protection.

   D. Seven-year-olds are not reliable witnesses of child abuse.

7. A realistic outcome criterion for a woman admitted with a broken collarbone caused by a husband with a history of violence would be that the woman might do which of the following?

   A. Fight back the next time he hurts her.

   B. Identify what she does that causes her husband to become violent.

   C. Leave the abusive man immediately and never see him again.

   D. State the names of two shelters she can go to when necessary.

8. The nurse caring for an abused child or abused woman should do which of the following?

   A. Allow the family members to remain alone together as much as possible, regardless of the situation, to facilitate family stability.

   B. Assume that the abuse was malicious and isolate the victim from family members.

   C. Refrain from becoming emotionally involved in the situation.

   D. Stay with the child or abused woman throughout the examination process and questioning sessions to offer needed support.

9. Which of the following is true about abuse?

   A. Neglect can be an unintentional form of child abuse.

   B. Psychological abuse is not as damaging as physical abuse.

   C. The goal of nursing care in abuse situations is to keep families together throughout therapy.

   D. Victims of abuse experience guilt only if they caused the abuser to become violent.

PART 2

Determine if the following nursing interventions are appropriate or inappropriate for a child or domestic abuse victim. Indicate your answer by placing an "A" or an "I" in the space provided.

1. _____ Inform the parents you suspect child abuse as soon as you note suspicious signs.

2. _____ Interview the victim in front of the abuser to make the abuser confess to the crime.

3. _____ Examine the child or suspected victim in a fully undressed state whenever possible.

4. _____ Protect the child's or victim's modesty as much as possible.

5. _____ Do not try to nurture the infant with failure to thrive since this will interfere with family-child bonding.

6. _____ Take photographs of injuries and bruises.

7. _____ Suspect overprotective partners of rape victims of being potential abusers.

8. _____ Write the exact words spoken by abuse victims and others describing the situation in the patient care chart.

9. _____ Encourage victims to talk about the abuse or rape to help them begin to work through it.

10. _____ Instruct women that the examination after the rape will be the only one she will have to submit to.

PART 3: CASE STUDY

Alissa, age 26, appears in your emergency room with her 4-year-old daughter, Daisy. She states, "He's hurting her. See, he's made her bleed." Alissa is pointing at Daisy's underpants, which are soiled with a dark-red stain.

1. What would your initial actions be?

2. How would you proceed in your care planning for Daisy?

3. What issues might you need to address with Alissa if the "he" she referred to was Alissa's husband or live-in boyfriend? If "he" is Alissa's father (Daisy's grandfather)?

■ Section Four: Inquiry and Exploration

PART 1: CRITICAL INQUIRY EXERCISES

1. Describe your feelings about a report of rape made by a female child 5 years of age who says, "Daddy hurt me."

2. What would your response be to a male adolescent who reports that his coach sexually abused him, or to a wife who says her husband raped her?

PART 2: CRITICAL EXPLORATION EXERCISES

Visit a rape crisis center in your neighborhood. Note three activities performed by the nurse in that setting.

CHAPTER 56

Nursing Care of the Family Coping With Long-Term or Terminal Illness

CHAPTER OVERVIEW

Chapter 56 discusses the physiologic and emotional concerns related to caring for a family coping with a long-term or fatal illness. The emotional effects of chronic and terminal illness on the entire family as well as on the nursing care provider are reviewed. The use of the nursing process to plan and provide care for the family involved with long-term or terminal illness is explored.

LEARNING OBJECTIVES

After mastering the contents of this chapter, you should be able to:

1. Describe common concerns of parents of children with a long-term or fatal illness.

2. Assess adjustment of the child and family with a long-term or terminal illness.

3. Use the nursing process to identify and address nursing diagnoses for the child with a chronic or fatal illness.

4. Identify National Health Goals related to children with long-term or fatal illnesses that nurses could be instrumental in helping the nation achieve.

5. Use critical thinking to analyze ways that nursing care of chronically ill or dying children can be more family-centered.

6. Synthesize knowledge of long-term and fatal illness in children with the nursing process to achieve quality child health nursing care.

KEY TERMS

anticipatory grief
death
grief process
vulnerable children

▪ Section One:
Identification of Key Terms and Concepts

PART 1

Match the terms in Part A with a definition or related statement from Part B. Place the letter corresponding to the answer in the space provided.

PART A

1. _____ Infant

2. _____ Toddler

3. _____ Preschooler

4. _____ School-ager

5. _____ Adolescent

PART B

A. Early in this stage view death as temporary, later realize death is final; focus on how they will cope without parents

B. See death as sleep and fear separation more than death

C. Have no understanding of their impending death; comfort and security are their main focus

D. Have adult concerns of death but view themselves as basically indestructible; need to remain as active as possible

E. May have viewed the death of a relative but do not understand or relate this to their own death; need to maintain routines

PART 2

Match each term in Part A with its definition or related statement in Part B. Place the letter corresponding to the answer in the space provided.

PART A

1. _____ Anticipatory grief

2. _____ Bargaining stage

3. _____ Depression

4. _____ Denial stage

5. _____ Anger stage

6. _____ Hospice

7. _____ Death

8. _____ Organ donation

9. _____ Autopsy

10. _____ Grief reaction

PART B

A. Defined by the absence of respirations, no heart sounds, absence of body movement or reflexes, and dilated fixed pupils

B. Is experienced when news of chronic illness or impending death is received

C. May provide a comfort for parents to know a part of their child has helped another child to live

D. Parent may promise to do good deeds so the terminally ill child will get well

E. The nurse may be an ineffective caregiver when in this stage since problem-solving skills are impaired

F. Mandatory if homicide, suicide, or harmful death is suspected

G. A third opinion regarding the disease or prognosis may be requested

H. Provides an option for children to die in a homelike setting

I. Parents begin to really think about the child's impending death

J. Parents may criticize the nurse or scold the child frequently

■ Section Two:
Short Answer and Completion Exercises

PART 1

Complete the following fill-in-the-blank exercises.

1. People cope with situations depending on _____ , _____ , and

   _____ .

2. A client or family's ability to use health care resources depends on

   _____ _____ , _____ , _____ , _____ ,

   and _____ .

3. Two of the reactions a nurse may have to the terminal illness of a child include

   _____ and _____ .

4. Nurses can help the nation meet National Health Goals related to chronic

   illness in children by educating women to seek care for themselves during

   pregnancy so _____ _____ are reduced, and seek _____

   for their children so diseases that can lead to long-term disability can be

   prevented.

PART 2

Complete the following short answer exercises.

1. Briefly compare the effects a chronic illness such as diabetes might have on a family with the effects of a chronic illness such as muscular dystrophy.

2. Discuss how the age of the parents might affect their ability to care for a disabled child.

3. Why would healthy parents of a chronically ill or disabled child need to have a will prepared?

4. How might evaluating the plan of care for a family with a terminal child after the child's death be beneficial for a nurse?

5. List three of the seven approaches to communicating with dying children.

_____   _____

_____

■ Section Three:
Critical Thinking for Application of Essential Concepts

PART 1

Circle the letter corresponding to the appropriate answer.

1. Bobby, age 10, has a diagnosis of juvenile diabetes. His mother has expressed plans to tutor Bobby at home and design a comfortable, quiet life to help him cope with his condition. Which of the following nursing diagnoses would best address this situation?

    A. Altered maternal bonding related to chronic illness

    B. Grieving related to loss of child's expected activity level

    C. High risk for altered growth and development related to lack of age-appropriate stimulation

    D. Ineffective family coping, disabling, related to parent's inability to accept child's illness

2. Polly, age 5, is admitted to the hospital with cystic fibrosis and pneumonia. Polly's mother tells the nurse that Polly must have pulmonary therapy before breakfast in order to eat a good meal. The nurse should respond in which of the following ways?

   A. Assure Polly's mother that the hospital staff is very competent and will take good care of the child.

   B. Inform Polly's mother of the visiting hours and insist she go home and rest since Polly is in good hands.

   C. Listen to the mother and note the schedule and procedures that Polly is accustomed to at home.

   D. Nod, and after the mother has gone plan Polly's care according to the hospital schedule.

3. Mr. and Mrs. Peters have a 4-year-old son, Bryan, who has been diagnosed with a terminal illness. The nurse would be concerned if which of the following plans were made by the family?

   A. Arrangements were being made to find a consistent sitter who could care for Bryan while Mrs. Peters works 4 hours a day.

   B. Mr. Peters states he plans to stay home with Bryan in the evenings so that Mrs. Peters can go to her exercise class.

   C. Mrs. Peters states she intends to care for Bryan around the clock and will need no assistance from anyone.

   D. The Peters family intends to take Bryan home and care for him there so he will die surrounded by family members.

4. David, 14, has leukemia and is in the hospital for the fourth time. When assessing a mother to determine if she is progressing through the stages of grief over her teenage son's terminal illness, the nurse would find which of the following to be signs of maladaptive coping?

   A. David's mother seems very sad at times and occasionally walks out of his room crying.

   B. David's mother shows the same signs of denial she showed when he was admitted to the hospital the first time.

   C. David's mother speaks of how good a son he was and how she is really going to miss him.

   D. David's mother spends a lot of time with David and brings him all his favorite foods from home.

5. The nurse notes that a terminally ill child's parents are not visiting very frequently or providing needed support. Which of the following could the nurse do?

   A. Call the parents in and have them explain to the child why they are not visiting as often as they should.

   B. Spend as much time with the child as possible, recognizing that the parents may need to withdraw temporarily to cope.

   C. Tell the child it is good to have time alone to think about death and to prepare for this new experience.

   D. Warn the parents that if they do not visit the child frequently now, they may experience intense guilt feelings after death.

PART 2: CASE STUDY

Patricia, age 10, is involved in an automobile accident that results in facial scarring. Her parents arrived an hour ago and have been told that plastic surgery will help but cannot fully repair the damage to Patricia's face.

1. What reactions might you expect from Patricia when she discovers the condition of her face? What factors might affect the extent and demonstration of her grief?

2. How might Patricia's reaction differ from that of a 14- or 15-year-old girl?

■ Section Four: Inquiry and Exploration

PART 1: CRITICAL INQUIRY EXERCISES

1. How might you feel if a patient you cared for over several weeks died on your day off? How would those feelings differ, if at all, if the patient was elderly and terminally ill; a young adult automobile accident victim; a child; or recovering well when you left the day before?

2. How would your approach differ, if at all, when providing care for the family members of a patient who died suddenly, and providing care for family members of a patient who died after a long hospitalization during which the patient wasted away and experienced pain?

PART 2: CRITICAL EXPLORATION EXERCISES

1. Spend a day with a chronically ill child and his or her family. Record interactions and determine if any maladaptive coping behaviors are present.

2. Spend a day with a terminally ill child and his or her family. Note the family dynamics (reactions of the child and parents). Record your reaction to the situation, the child, and the family.

Answers

Chapter 1

SECTION ONE
PART 1

1. D   2. G   3. C   4. H   5. B   6. A   7. E   8. F

PART 2

1. B   2. C   3. F   4. D   5. A

SECTION TWO
PART 1

1. Any two of the following would be accurate: families are smaller in size; single parents are increasing in number; an increasing number of mothers work outside the home; families are more mobile, with increased number of homeless women and children; abuse is more common; families are more health conscious; and health care must respect cost containment (see Table 1-3 in text for possible implications).
2. Nursing staff will be required to provide intensive health teaching with follow-up by home care nurses. Patients and parents must be prepared to recognize danger signs that warrant immediate attention and to respond appropriately. Parents should be allowed to do as much for the child/newborn as they wish to prepare them to care for the child/newborn upon discharge.
3. The following are methods for promoting empowerment: addressing the client by name; regarding parents as important participants in their child's health by keeping the child and parents informed of the child's status and including them in the decision-making process; and making each client feel important.

PART 2

1. prematurity; low birthweight; congenital anomalies, respiratory distress syndrome, sudden infant death syndrome
2. before; care for
3. neonatal nurse practitioner
4. scope

SECTION THREE

1. B   2. D   3. D   4. B   5. C   6. B

Chapter 2

SECTION ONE

1. e   2. a   3. d   4. b   5. c

SECTION TWO
PART 1

1. structure; function
2. orientation; procreation
3. foster
4. communal
5. lesbian and gay

PART 2

1. physical maintenance
2. socialization of family members

3. allocation of resources
4. maintenance of order
5. division of labor
6. reproduction, recruitment, and release of family members
7. placement of member into the larger society
8. maintenance of motivation and morale

SECTION THREE

1. C   2. A   3. C   4. B

Chapter 3

SECTION ONE

1. b   2. e   3. f   4. d   5. a   6. c

SECTION TWO

1. Hispanic
2. Chinese American
3. Vietnamese American; spirit

SECTION THREE

PART 1

1. B   2. A   3. D   4. C

Chapter 4

SECTION ONE
PART 1

1. e   2. i   3. d   4. f   5. k   6. b   7. g   8. h   9. j   10. c   11. a

PART 2

1. a   2. g   3. c   4. e   5. f   6. h   7. d   8. b

PART 3

1. b   2. a   3. d   4. c

PART 4

1. F   2. T

SECTION TWO

1. gonad
2. menopause
3. androgenic hormones
4. thelarche
5. homologous
6. gynecology

SECTION THREE
PART 1

1. D   2. C   3. A

Chapter 5

SECTION ONE

1. c   2. e   3. d   4. b   5. a   6. f

SECTION TWO
PART 1

1. Nausea, vomiting, acne, monilial vaginal infections, mild hypertension, weight gain
2. Estrogen, the content of the pill, suppresses the follicle stimulating hormone (FSH), luteinizing hormone (LH), and gonadotropic hormone. The progesterone constituent decreases the permeability of cervical mucus, limiting sperm mobility and access to the ovum. Progesterone interferes with endometrial proliferation, making implantation unlikely.
3. The "mini pill" differs from the traditional oral contraceptive in that it is composed of progesterone only. Ovulation occurs, but implantation will not.
4. IUDs are rarely selected as a method of contraception for the adolescent girl. They are not recommended for women who have not been pregnant or who have multiple sex partners. It is unlikely that the adolescent would fit this criterion. Spermicides: This barrier method is widely used by the adolescent population. It is economical and requires no parental consent. However, the method has a conception rate of 20%. The adolescent tends to engage in sexual activity without tradition. Coitus is often hurried and takes place in settings that tend to make the girl feel awkward when wanting to use a contraceptive product. Condoms: Adolescents should be cautioned carefully about the use of condoms. They are most effective when applied before any penile-vulvar contact. The self-lubricated type breaks less frequently. The condom should fit loosely enough to allow the penis tip to collect the ejaculate without undue pressure. Condom efficiency is lessened by body heat when carried for some time in pockets and wallets. The use of a vaginally inserted preparation enhances the efficiency of the condom.

PART 2

IUD: Description: Small plastic object inserted into the vagina; physiologic effect: Interferes with the ability of an ovum to develop; effect on future pregnancy: If pregnancy is suspected, the physician should be notified; the IUD is removed vaginally if a woman becomes pregnant

Barrier methods: Description: Spermicidal jellies, creams, and gels inserted into the vagina before coitus; physiologic effect: Change the vaginal pH to an acid level not conducive for the life of sperm. Sponge impregnated with spermicide creates foaming action in vagina to protect against invading spermatozoa; effect on future pregnancy: No harm to the fetus if pregnancy occurs

Diaphragm: Description: A circular rubber disk that fits over the cervix to form a barrier against the entrance of spermatozoa; physiologic effect: Impedes the passage of spermatozoa from the vagina to the cervix after coitus; effect on future pregnancy: No risk or harm to fetus

Condom: Description: A rubber or synthetic sheath that is placed over the erect penis before coitus; most effective when treated with nonoxynol-9; physiologic effect: Prevents pregnancy because the spermatozoa are deposited in the tip of the condom instead of in the vagina; effect on future pregnancy: No risk to fetus

SECTION THREE
PART 1

1. B   2. A   3. B   4. B

Chapter 6

SECTION ONE

1. G   2. H   3. D   4. J   5. A   6. C   7. I   8. B   9. E   10. F

SECTION TWO
PART 1

1. relief; stoic acceptance; grief
2. surrogate mother
3. gender/genetic preselection
4. artificial insemination
5. in vitro

PART 2

1. Decrease frequency of coitus/intercourse; wear clothing that does not restrict or overheat the scrotum; avoid frequent use of hot baths.
2. Couples experiencing infertility may experience fear and anxiety regarding the outcome of the testing, frustration and disappointment related to the time and strict routines involved in the testing process, and loss of self-esteem and fear of loss of their partner on learning of the infertility.
3. Any of the following would be accurate: (1) childless living allows a couple the opportunity for career growth, (2) they can travel more, (3) they can pursue hobbies, (4) continuance of education is easier, (5) childless living allows couples to make a more personal contribution to society.

SECTION THREE
PART 1

1. B   2. C   3. C

PART 2

1. A   2. I   3. I   4. A   5. I

Chapter 7

SECTION ONE
PART 1

1. F   2. D   3. I   4. A   5. H   6. C   7. E   8. J   9. B   10. G

PART 2

1. C   2. A   3. B, D   4. G, H, E   5. B   6. I, E   7. B, D

SECTION TWO
PART 1

1. Genetic testing allows the couple to make informed choices about future reproduction.
2. If the disease is dominantly inherited, 3 of 4 children could inherit the disease; if the disease is recessively inherited, 1 of 4 children could inherit the disease (see text: Fig. 7-2).
3. Any two of the following: reassure people who are concerned that their children will inherit a disorder that their fears are groundless (if what they are concerned about is not an inherited disorder); allow people who are affected by inherited disorders to make informed choices about future reproduction; educate people about inherited disorders and the process of inheritance; offer support by skilled health care professionals to people who are affected by genetic illness.
4. In both situations, the couple would be too emotionally shocked and grief-stricken to receive genetic counseling.

PART 2

1. inform; inherit
2. legal; ethical
3. self-esteem; support

SECTION THREE
PART 1

1. B   2. A   3. D   4. B   5. B   6. C   7. C   8. B

Chapter 8

SECTION ONE

1. G   2. D   3. J   4. A   5. I   6. E   7. H   8. B   9. F   10. C

SECTION TWO
PART 1

End of 8 gestation weeks: Heart has septum and valves. Facial features are definitely discernible.

End of 12 gestation weeks: Nail beds forming on toes and fingers; tooth buds present; heart sounds audible by Doppler instrument

End of 16 gestation weeks: Formation of lanugo; liver and pancreas are functioning; fetus demonstrates swallowing reflex

End of 20 gestation weeks: Quickening; beginning of vernix caseosa

End of 24 gestation weeks: Average weight is 550 g; passive antibody transfer from mother to fetus

End of 28 gestation weeks: Average weight is 1,200 g; lung alveoli begin maturing with surfactant

End of 32 gestation weeks: Average weight is 1,600 g; assumes delivery position; store iron

End of 36 gestation weeks: Additional deposits of subcutaneous fat and lanugo start to diminish

End of 40 gestation weeks: Fetus kicks actively; fetal hemoglobin begins to convert to adult hemoglobin; lightening occurs

PART 2

1. Selected osmosis through chorionic villi

SECTION THREE
PART 1

1. B   2. B   3. B   4. A   5. C

Chapter 9

SECTION ONE

1. b   2. c   3. a   4. b   5. a   6. c   7. b   8. a   9. b   10. B   11. b

SECTION TWO
PART 1

1. The nurse can play an important role in promoting health during pregnancy by providing preconception counseling and particularly by being certain that adolescents receive counseling in nutrition and safe/safer sex practices.

2. The lateral recumbent position would help prevent pressure on the vena cava that could impair circulation, and also help assist the kidneys to function at maximum efficiency.

3. The kidneys are taxed heavily to filter an increased blood volume. The glomerular filtration rate is increased, filtering glucose faster than the renal tubules can reabsorb it and therefore accidentally spilling glucose into the urine. In addition, lactose, the sugar of breast milk, will be spilled in the urine during pregnancy.

4. After confirmation of pregnancy, most women are more conscious about their diets, the use of over-the-counter medicines, and cigarette smoking. Also, if the woman desires to voluntarily terminate the pregnancy, the risk of complications from an abortion is minimized.

PART 2

The following changes are most common, see text for others.

1. Gastrointestinal system: displacement of the stomach and intestines, giving rise to heartburn, constipation, and flatulence; "morning sickness," theoretically due to decreased glucose levels from fetal consumption; after 3 months will experience increased appetite; hyperptyalism (increased saliva production) due to high estrogen levels
2. Urinary system: an increase in body water to 7.5 liters to help increase circulatory blood volume and provide nutrients to the fetus; increase in glomerular filtration rate and the renal plasma flow to meet the increased needs of the circulatory system; increased bladder capacity, with urinary frequency noted in first and third trimesters due to pressure from uterus
3. Skeletal system: change of posture to center the mass of pregnancy, creating lordosis and backache; softening of the pelvic ligaments and joints
4. Endocrine system: formulation of the placenta as an endocrine gland that produces estrogen and progesterone, relaxin, human chorionic gonadotropin, and human placental lactogen; an increase in the parathyroid's size and function to supply additional regulation of calcium; late in pregnancy, pituitary gland produces oxytocin and prolactin; pancreas decreases insulin in early pregnancy and increases insulin in third trimester; thyroid gland slightly enlarges with increased thyroid hormone production
5. Respiratory system: changes in CO_2 level described as a chronic respiratory alkalosis fully compensated by a chronic metabolic acidosis; marked congestion or "stuffiness" of the nasopharynx in response to increased estrogen levels; hyperventilation and increased total ventilatory capacity to help handle the extra load of CO_2 produced by the fetus

SECTION THREE
PART 1

1. D   2. C   3. B   4. B   5. A

Chapter 10

SECTION ONE
Part 1

1. T   2. F   3. F   4. F   5. T

SECTION TWO
Part 1

1. Gynecoid: well-rounded inlet, wide pubic arch
2. Anthropoid: transverse diameter is narrow and anteroposterior diameter of the inlet is larger than normal
3. Platypelloid: oval-shaped inlet, smoothly curved
4. Android: pubic arch forms an acute angle, narrowing lower dimensions of the pelvis

Part 2

1. Endocervical: use a wet saline cotton swab applicator and insert it through the speculum into the os of the cervix. Rotate clockwise and counterclockwise. Place on laboratory slide.
2. Cervical os: press uneven end of supplied spatula on the os, rotate, and scrape cells in a circular motion. Place on laboratory slide.
3. Vaginal: place cotton swab applicator just below the cervix, rolling gently to obtain secretions. Place on laboratory slide.

SECTION THREE

Part 1

1. C   2. C   3. B   4.D   5 .B   6. C

Chapter 11

SECTION ONE

1. I   2. F   3. G   4. A   5. H   6. B   7. J   8. E   9. C   10. D

SECTION TWO
PART 1

1. teratogens; abnormalities in physical or emotional health
2. teaching
3. Any five of the following would be accurate: breast tenderness, constipation, nausea, vomiting, pyrosis, fatigue, palmar erythema, muscle cramps, hypotension, varicosities, hemorrhoids, urinary frequency, heart palpitations, abdominal discomfort, leukorrhea and pruritus.
4. metal; chemical; radiation; hypothermia, hyperthermia

PART 2

1. Bathing: tub baths are permitted unless membranes are ruptured, cervical dilation is present, or balance is disturbed. Breast care: firm bra with wide straps, wash colostrum away with clean water, use pads inside bra to keep nipples dry and change frequently, and nipple-rolling exercise if breast-feeding is intended. Perineal hygiene: Douching is discouraged, but with vinegar solution and gravity, douche may be used. Dressing: common sense and comfort, light girdle for support, large-sized bra, avoid restrictive clothing. Sexual activity: permitted as tolerated, except when membranes have ruptured or vaginal spotting is noted; if history of spontaneous abortion, refrain from sex until after the time of prior abortion; use of condom with nonmonogamous partners, use caution with oral-genital contact. Exercise: individualized, moderate activity, walking encouraged, jogging or body contact sports may be contraindicated. Sleep: increased amounts encouraged, relaxation exercises, afternoon naps in late pregnancy. Travel: no restrictions in early pregnancy, late in pregnancy arrange for emergency care in case of early labor; frequent stretching on long trips.
2. Lightening, settling of the fetal head into the inlet of the true pelvis; show, the release of the cervical plug that formed during pregnancy; rupture of the membranes, gush of amniotic fluid from the vagina; excess energy, the body's physiologic preparation for labor; and uterine contractions usually begin labor.
3. Refer to Table 11-1 of the text.
4. Refer to Focus on Family Empowerment in the text; any two instructions in each category are correct.
5. Anxiety produces physiologic changes leading to vasoconstriction and decreased fetal blood supply, and possibly to preterm labor.

SECTION THREE

1. B   2. A   3. B   4. A   5. C   6. C   7. B

Chapter 12

SECTION ONE

1. d   2. e   3. b   4. i   5. a   6. h   7. j   8. c   9. f   10. g

SECTION TWO
PART 1

1. 11.2 kg to 16 kg (25 to 40 lb)
2. quality
3. 1,500
4. D; B12; calcium

PART 2

1. Inadequate maternal dietary intake could result in fetal deprivation with premature birth,

a stillborn infant, functional immaturity, or congenital birth defects.

2. High parity, short intervals between pregnancies, or rigorous dieting for weight loss may deplete nutritional reserves (see text for additional factors).

3. Foods with caffeine should be avoided because caffeine stimulates the central nervous system and is associated with low birthweight. Artificial sweeteners should be avoided as much as possible, since safety is not completely established; saccharine is eliminated slowly from the fetus.

4. Protein: Source: meat, eggs, milk. Significance: supplies needed B vitamins (B_{12}) and essential amino acids. Calcium: Source: milk, milk products. Significance: necessary for fetal skeletal and tooth formation. Fat: Source: vegetable oils are preferred. Significance: supplies essential fatty acid needed for new cell growth. Folic acid: Source: fresh fruits and vegetables. Significance: necessary for red blood cell formation. Iodine: Source: iodized salt, seafood. Significance: essential for the formation of the thyroid hormone thyroxine. Iron: Source: organ meats, eggs, green leafy vegetables, whole-grain breads, dried fruit. Significance: needed to build hemoglobin and increased red cell volume.

SECTION THREE
PART 1

1. A   2. C   3. A   4. C   5. B

Chapter 13

SECTION ONE

1. d   2. f   3. b   4. a   5. e   6. c

SECTION TWO
PART 1

1. cleansing breath
2. gate control
3. psychosexual method
4. effleurage
5. Kegel exercises
6. psychoprophylaxis

PART 2

Hospital Settings: Attended by skilled professionals during labor, birth, and the postpartal period; encouraged to be prepared to control the discomfort of birthing through nonmedication measures; encouraged to consider breast-feeding; emergency care and extended high-risk care are immediately available. Mother does not feel totally in control of the birthing process and there is separation from family.

Alternative Birth Center: Extended high-risk care is easily arranged. A minimum of analgesia and anesthesia is provided. The woman may be fatigued following birth, and she must independently monitor her postpartal status.

Home Birth: The woman has more control over the childbirth experience and may avoid nosocomial infections; she has the greatest freedom to express her individuality, and there is no separation from family; allows for family integrity. Possible interference with taking-in phase; woman must independently monitor her postpartal status.

PART 3

1. If the peripheral nerves associated with an injury at the site are stimulated, the nerve fibers at that injury site transmit less effectively. Therefore, effleurage is considered effective in the active state of labor.

2. If brain cells that register pain are all preoccupied with stimuli other than pain, these cells will not register pain. Therefore, focusing on other stimuli will divert attention and reduce pain.

3. Pain impulses to the brain are enhanced in the presence of anxiety. Reducing anxiety will reduce pain perception.

SECTION THREE

1. B   2. A   3. B   4. C   5. B

Chapter 14

SECTION ONE
PART 1

1. C   2. J   3. F   4. A   5. K   6. H   7. I   8. G   9. B   10. L

PART 2

1. C   2. D   3. E   4. F   5. B   6. A

SECTION TWO
PART 1

1. Refer to Box 14-1 in the text for examples.
2. Pregnancy results in dilated ureters and stasis of urine, which predisposes a woman to urinary tract infection.
3. Diet: 1,800- to 2,200-calorie diet, evenly distributed over three meals and three snacks. Exercise: begin exercise regimen before pregnancy, maintain consistent daily exercise, eat a protein or complex carbohydrate snack before exercise. Insulin: dosage and type may need adjustment-less early in pregnancy, more late in pregnancy. Glucose monitoring: blood testing is preferred; use milk to treat hypoglycemia.
4. Any four of the following would be accurate. Candidiasis: can cause candidal infection or thrush in the newborn during the first trimester. Trichomoniasis: associated with preterm labor; Flagyl is teratogenic. Bacterial vaginosis: associated with amniotic fluid infection and perhaps preterm labor. *Chlamydia trachomatis:* associated with premature rupture of membranes, preterm labor, conjunctivitis, or pneumonia. Syphilis: associated with preterm labor, stillbirth, or congenital anomalies. Herpes simplex 2: congenital infection. Gonorrhea: associated with spontaneous abortion, preterm delivery, eye infection, and blindness. Group B streptococci: neonatal infection with pneumonia or meningitis. Human immunodeficiency virus: may be passed to fetus/infant.
5. Refer to Focus on Family Teaching in the text. Possible answers include: Home: do not use step stools or ladders, keep small items out of the pathway, no throw rugs, be cautious using the tub, do not overload electrical circuits, don't smoke (particularly not in bed), have good lighting when taking medications. Work: avoid toxic substances, avoid fatigue, do not stand for long periods. Auto: use seat belts at all times, do not ride with individuals who are impaired due to drugs or alcohol.
6. If victim is standing or lying, fists should be positioned in mediastinal region. Pressure should be applied straight back, if victim is standing, or straight down, if victim is lying.

PART 2

1. Poor placental perfusion
2. Stasis of blood; hypercoagulability; blood vessel damage
3. Nasopharyngitis: Maternal effect/treatment: breathing difficulty, no treatment. Fetal effect/treatment: none documented. Asthma: Maternal effect: condition may improve; hypoxia, if attack occurs. Fetal effect: hypoxia, if attack occurs. Treatment for maternal and fetal effect: beta-adrenergic agonists can depress labor and must be tapered. Pneumonia: Maternal effect/treatment: hypoxia, preterm labor, oxygen therapy may be needed. Fetal effect/treatment: Hypoxia, oxygen needed, preterm birth. Tuberculosis: Maternal effect/treatment: may be reactivated by pressure on the lungs, may delay maternal contact with infant, TB medications are taken during pregnancy. Fetal effect/treatment: may be transmitted in utero or after birth; maternal treatment.

SECTION THREE
PART 1

1. D   2. B   3. A   4. D   5. A   6. D   7. B   8. A   9. A
10. D   11. B   12. C   13. C   14. C   15. B   16. C   17. D   18. B   19. A

Chapter 15

SECTION ONE
PART 1
1. D 2. G 3. F 4. I 5. L 6. H 7. M 8. A 9. E 10. C

PART 2
1. C 2. A 3. B 4. C 5. B 6. A

SECTION TWO
PART 1
1. spontaneous miscarriage
2. ectopic pregnancy
3. HELLP syndrome
4. mild preeclampsia
5. hydramnios

PART 2
1. The time during pregnancy at which bleeding occurs helps in the identification of the cause of the bleeding.
2. A woman with an ectopic pregnancy may experience the same initial symptoms of early pregnancy. However, if tubal rupture occurs, the woman may experience a sharp, stabbing lower abdominal pain; vaginal spotting; a bluish umbilicus; and possibly signs of shock.
3. In placenta previa the placenta is implanted in the lower part of the uterus, whereas in abruptio placenta correct implantation is present but sudden placental separation from the uterus, with bleeding, is noted.
4. Heparin is used in DIC to stop the clotting cascade and stop blood coagulation so that coagulation factors will be released to be available for use throughout the body.
5. A woman with multiple gestation may be instructed to do the following: maintain bed rest the last 2 to 3 months of pregnancy; refrain from coitus during the last 2 to 3 months of pregnancy; plan extra rest time during the day; eat six small meals per day instead of three large ones; report any abnormal bleeding or swelling, since the risk for eclampsia, hydramnios, placenta previa, and anemia is higher in multiple gestation. Counseling to help the woman work through two role changes instead of one should also be a part of the teaching plan.

SECTION THREE
1. C 2. D 3. D 4. A 5. C 6. C 7. C 8. B 9. D 10. A 11. C 12. B 13. C

Chapter 16

SECTION ONE
1. b 2. a 3. e 4. d

SECTION TWO
PART 1
1. family routines
2. privacy; confidentiality
3. leave; call; community emergency number
4. expected; they can expect

PART 2
1. Nurses can encourage women to seek prenatal care and can educate women about the signs and symptoms of preterm labor so women can get help at a point at which labor can be halted.
2. Client: health history, physical exam, mental and psychological assessments (if she is resting, how she occupies her time), that self-assessments are being made accurately, and

that she knows to keep health care appointments and has transportation. Environment: safety of house for home care; presence of adequate water, heat, and refrigeration; if rodents or insects are in the home.

3. Follow-up visits are planned depending on each woman's individual circumstances and the amount of health education and further supervision needed.

SECTION THREE
PART 1

1. B   2. C   3. D   4. A   5. D

Chapter 17

SECTION ONE
PART 1

1. E   2. F   3. D   4. J   5. C   6. I   7. H   8. A   9. B   10. G

PART 2

1. B, C, E, F
2. B, C, D, E, F
3. B, C, E, G
4. B, C, E, F, G
5. A, B, C, E, F

SECTION TWO
PART 1

1. Early age of menarche in girls, an increase in the rate of sexual activity among teenagers, and a lack of knowledge of (or inability to use) contraceptive information among sexually active teenagers and desire by teens to have a baby.
2. Any three of the following would be correct: pregnancy-induced hypertension, iron deficiency anemia, premature labor, preterm birth with low-birthweight infant, postpartal hemorrhage, and cephalopelvic disproportion.
3. emancipated minor

PART 2

1. The nurse can teach adolescents about the dangers of substance abuse and the complications, both psychological and physical, of teenage pregnancy. In addition, nurses can research effective birth control measures for adolescents (that they might actually use).
2. The nurse has a legal obligation to help devise a safe plan of care for the child while protecting the mentally retarded mother's right to maintain control of her child.
3. Any of the following would be accurate: fear of discovery and being reported to authorities for drug abuse, need for frequent drug doses and inability to wait for services, insufficient finances to support both her drug habit and medical care and nutritious food.

SECTION THREE
PART 1

1. A   2. C   3. B   4. A   5. A   6. A   7. B   8. D   9. D   10. A

Chapter 18

SECTION ONE
PART 1

1. d   2. k   3. h   4. b   5. a   6. c   7. f   8. e   9. g   10. j

PART 2

1. e   2. d   3. f   4. c   5. a

SECTION TWO
PART 1

1. uterus; cervix; vagina; external perineum
2. preparatory
3. Any three of the following are correct: ripening of the cervix, increased activity level, Braxton Hicks contractions, lightening, show, and rupture of the membranes.
4. of appropriate size and in an advantageous position and presentation; of adequate size and contour; adequate to expel the fetus
5. inspection; palpation; vaginal examination; fetal heart tones; sonography
6. ripening
7. temperature
8. minus (negative); plus (positive)

PART 2

1. Any three of the following would be correct: uterine muscle stretching, pressure on cervix, oxytocin stimulation, change in ratio of estrogen and progesterone, placental age and deterioration, rising fetal cortisol levels, and fetal membrane production of prostaglandin.
2. Diaphoresis serves to cool and limit warming of the woman through the evaporation process.
3. Labor is longer due to ineffective descent of the fetus, ineffective dilation of the cervix, and irregular and weak uterine contractions.
4. Leopold's maneuvers are a systematic method of observation and palpation to determine fetal presentation and position. Four maneuvers are performed with the woman in a supine position with her knees flexed and her bladder empty. (Refer to text Fig. 18-1 for description of each maneuver.)
5. Labor can result in emotional distress, fatigue, and fear in the woman. The nurse should provide culturally sensitive support and stress-reduction measures, promote the presence of a significant other, explain all actions, and not be judgmental or have high expectations of the woman's performance.
6. The mother's pulse and blood pressure both increase during contractions. The fetal pulse may slow slightly during contractions.
7. The father or significant other can provide an important support to the mother during the labor process and may serve as a labor coach.
8. Fetal tachycardia indicates fetal distress (severe-due to hypoxia, maternal fever, drugs, fetal arrhythmia, or maternal anemia or hyperthyroidism). Fetal bradycardia (severe) signifies fetal hypoxia. Late deceleration suggests uteroplacental insufficiency or decreased uterine blood flow during contractions. Variable pattern indicates compression of the cord. Sinusoidal pattern indicates fetal anemia or hypoxia.

PART 3
Refer to page 473 of the text to check position descriptions.

SECTION THREE
PART 1

1. B	2. D	3. C	4. D	5. B	6. D	7. B	8. A	9. C	10. C
11. D	12. B	13. A	14. C	15. B	16. C	17. B			

Chapter 19

SECTION ONE

1. I	2. C	3. G	4. J	5. E	6. B	7. A	8. D	9. F	10. H

SECTION TWO
PART 1

1. enduring a painful labor
2. educating women about the advantages of prepared childbirth; helping women to use breathing patterns or other comfort techniques during labor so that they need a minimum

of analgesia and anesthesia; conscientious monitoring of women who receive analgesics and anesthesia during labor and birth

3. anoxia; stretching of the cervix and perineum
4. systemic; T10; L1
5. relax; systemic; contractions; effort

PART 2

1. Knowledge allows the woman to make the best choices for herself and her child; it also decreases fear and anxiety related to the labor experience.
2. Knowledge reduces anxiety and decreases the amount of pain medication required.
3. Pain medications given too early in the labor experience tend to slow or even stop contractions, which will delay dilation of the cervix and prolong labor. Once labor is well under way, however, pain medication could speed the progress of labor because the woman is able to work with, not against, contractions.
4. The significant other could provide support and decrease the woman's anxiety and pain.

PART 3

1. no
2. yes
3. no
4. yes
5. yes
6. yes

SECTION THREE
PART 1

1. B   2. B   3. C   4. A   5. C

Chapter 20

SECTION ONE
Part 1

1. B   2. C   3. D   4. A

Part 2

1. T   2. F   3. F   4. F

SECTION TWO

1. 300; 500; 500; 1000
2. poor nutritional status, age variations, poor general health, fluid and electrolyte imbalances, fear
3. A well-informed support person will be able to help minimize the client's experiences of anxiety.
4. A sonogram aids in locating the placenta to avoid an accidental incision of this organ during the surgical procedure.
5. Urinary output must be assessed to determine the presence of urinary retention, overextension of bladder capacity, and potential for permanent bladder damage, and to avoid interference with uterine contractions that may lead to postpartal hemorrhage. Voiding also provides evidence of adequate urinary and circulatory function.
6. Pneumonia: pain minimizes activity, allowing secretions in lung to pool. Pain increases when performing respiratory toileting exercise. Thrombophlebitis: pain discourages walking, leading to venous stasis and poor circulation of the femoral veins. Interference with maternal-infant bonding: experiences of pain lessen tactile stimulation, which hampers the bonding process.
7. Transcutaneous electrical nerve stimulation (TENS): method of controlling pain sensation by use of electrodes on the skin to irritate or stimulate the large afferent (sensory) nerve fibers, which facilitates the gating theory. The unit is turned on and off by the patient. Patient-controlled analgesia (PCA): pain control device. Patient administers precalculated

dose of intravenous narcotic analgesic by pressing a button on a special pump. Pump features a "lock-out" setting to prevent drug overdose.

SECTION THREE
Part 1

1. B   2. D   3. C   4. A   5. A

Chapter 21

SECTION ONE
PART 1

1. H   2. I   3. E   4. J   5. G   6. C   7. A   8. D   9. B   10. F

PART 2

1. A   2. A   3. B   4. A   5. A   6. A   7. B

SECTION TWO
PART 1

1. pressure on the cord; cord compression; hypoxia/anoxia
2. knee-chest; Trendelenburg
3. Inertia; dysfunctional
4. Cesarean section
5. Pathologic retraction ring; rupture
6. heart; lung

PART 2

1. the force that propels the fetus (uterine contractions); the passenger (the fetus); the passageway (the birth canal)
2. fetal monitoring and uterine monitoring
3. hypotonic uterine contractions; hypertonic uterine contractions; uncoordinated contractions
4. prolonged latent phase; prolonged deceleration phase, prolonged active phase; prolonged descent
5. small infants (SGA); cord prolapse; cord compression, intracranial hemorrhage, abnormal fetal presentation
6. dysfunctional labor, higher risk of anoxia from prolapsed cord; traumatic injury to the aftercoming head, fracture of the spine or arm
7. breech; face; transverse lie; brow
8. antidiuresis leading to possible water intoxication; jaundice in the newborn
9. woman is unable to push with contractions; cessation of progress in the second stage of labor; fetus in abnormal position, or fetus is immature
10. complete; frank; double footing; single footing
11. premature rupture of membranes; fetal position other than cephalic; placenta previa; intrauterine tumors that prevent engagement; small fetus; cephalopelvic disproportion, hydramnios, and multiple gestation
12. multiple gestation, faulty presentation, previous uterine surgery; previous uterine tears; prolonged labor; excessive use of oxytocin; obstructed labor; traumatic maneuvers/forceps or traction.

SECTION THREE
PART 1

1. B   2. A   3. C.   4. A   5. C.   6. D

Chapter 22

SECTION ONE
PART 1

1. F   2. I   3. C   4. D   5. A   6. H   7. B   8. J   9. E   10. G

PART 2

1. C   2. A   3. E   4. F   5. B   6. D

SECTION TWO
PART 1

1. taking-in phase
2. lochia serosa
3. lactation
4. episiotomy
5. Kegel (perineal)

PART 2

1. During the taking-in phase the woman is passive and wishes to be ministered to; during the taking-hold phase the woman begins to initiate actions and takes more, but not all, responsibility for herself and her child; during the letting-go phase the woman redefines and assumes her new role.
2. Complete and partial. Advantages: Allows the father and mother more time to develop a relationship with the child; the bonding process occurs more rapidly; helps build confidence in childcare before discharge.
3. amount; consistency; pattern, odor; absence
4. known as baby blues, decrease in estrogen and progesterone that occurs after delivery of the placenta; evidenced by tearfulness, feeling of inadequacy, mood lability, anorexia, and sleep disturbance
5. A sitz bath supplies moist heat, which increases circulation to the perineum, thereby reducing edema, and promotes healing and comfort. An ice bag during the first 24 hours postpartum will aid in reducing edema and possible hematoma formation and promote healing and comfort.

PART 3

Fundus: immediately postpartum can be found halfway between the umbilicus and symphysis pubis; it will decrease one fingerbreadth per day from the umbilicus (1 cm/day in size) until no longer palpable.

Cervix: immediately after delivery is soft and malleable with the internal and external os open; 7 days postpartum the external os is narrowed to a pencil-sized opening and is firm. The external os assumes a permanent star- or slit-like pattern.

Vagina: the hymen is permanently torn, the vagina is soft with few rugae, a large diameter, and a thin wall early postpartum; the wall may thicken and involute to prepregnancy size by 6 weeks postpartum with exercise and if proper hormone release resumes.

Perineum: edematous and tender initially with ecchymotic portions; the labia minora and majora remain atropic and softened.

SECTION THREE

1. B   2. C   3. C   4. C   5. A   6. B   7. C   8. C   9. B
10. C   11. D   12. D   13. A   14. B   15. C   16. A   17. B   18. D

Chapter 23

SECTION ONE
PART 1

1. C   2. G   3. B   4. F   5. H   6. D   7. I   8. A   9. K   10. J

PART 2

1. T   2. F   3. F   4. F

SECTION TWO
PART 1

1. neonatal period
2. convection; conduction; radiation; evaporation
3. 120-140/minute
4. 30-50/minute

PART 2

1. habituation, orientation, motor maturity, self-quieting ability, social behavior, variation
2. Bottle-fed: stools are bright yellow, have a more foul odor. Breast-fed: stools are light yellow, sweet-smelling.
3. Neonates who have not passed a stool in 24 hours past birth should be evaluated for meconium ileus, imperforate anus, or bowel obstruction.
4. First period of reactivity: rapid heartbeat and respiration, alert behavior, searching activity. Second period of reactivity: slowing of respiration and heart rate, infant may sleep for as long as 90-minute intervals.
5. A child of 20 pounds or less should be placed with the seat facing the back of the car; car seat should have a five-point harness with broad straps; parents should not use sack sleepers or papoose clothing. Seat should face backward until the infant can sit without support (approximately 17 pounds). When the infant can sit without support, he or she may be transferred to a toddler car seat.
6. Hemorrhage, infection, or urethral fistula may occur. Nursing interventions: check frequently for bleeding; note state of healing at each diaper change; avoid restrictive clothing or lying on abdomen; give care instructions to parent.
7. Cold sores may be indicative of herpes simplex; the infant's immature immune system may render him or her vulnerable to a grave illness.

SECTION THREE
PART 1

1. A   2. D   3. C   4. C   5. B

Chapter 24

SECTION ONE
PART 1

1. B   2. N   3. E   4. O   5. H   6. C   7. A   8. F   9. I
10. G   11. D   12. L   13. M   14. J   15. K

PART 2

1. T   2. T   3. F   4. F   5. T   6. T   7. F   8. F

SECTION TWO

1. Breast; mammary
2. Delivery of the placenta; prolactin
3. sucking on the breast
4. anterior pituitary; prolactin
5. Oxytocin released may lead to the onset of preterm labor.

SECTION THREE
PART 1

1. B   2. A   3. C   4. C   5. D   6. A   7. C   8. D

Chapter 25

SECTION ONE
PART 1

1. E   2. G   3. A   4. D   5. F   6. C   7. B

PART 2

1. T   2. T   3. T   4. F

SECTION TWO
PART 1

1. uterine atony, lacerations, retained placental fragments, and disseminated intravascular coagulation
2. deficiency in clotting, caused by low level of fibrinogen
3. premature separation of the placenta, missed abortion, fetal death in utero
4. Signs of postpartal-induced hypertension are the same as those of prepartal hypertension: proteinuria, edema, and hypertension.

PART 2

1. When wiping from back to front, organisms may be brought forward from the rectum to the vagina or perineal site of injury.
2. weighing perineal pads before and after saturation
3. Notice the amount of lochia. Determine if bright-red blood continues to be a part of lochia from the placenta site.
4. Assess lochia for color, odor, amount. Assess uterus for tenderness, size, and consistency. Assess vital signs to support evaluation of other data.
5. Placenta may be classed as succenturiate placenta; sections of this type may remain following a delivery and need to be surgically removed.

SECTION THREE
PART 1

1. D   2. C   3. C   4. A   5. B   6. C

Chapter 26

SECTION ONE
PART 1

1. B   2. C   3. A

PART 2

1. E   2. C   3. D   4. A   5. B

PART 3

1. T   2. T   3. F   4. F

SECTION TWO
PART 1

1. During the first few seconds of life, infant takes several weak gasps of air and then immediately stops breathing.
2. Placenta received insufficient nutrients: partial placental separation leading to bleeding; infarction, fibrosis, and reduced placental surface for exchange. Inefficient transport of nutrients to the fetus: systemic diseases in the mother may cause decreased blood flow to the placenta. Lack of adequate nutrition: poor nutritional intake occurs in teen pregnancy.
3. Mechanical treatment for severe hypertension; blood is shunted by gravity from the right atrium to the ECMO machine for oxygenation and warming, then returned to the patient via catheter through the carotid to the aortic arch.

4. Vitamin E is necessary for the formulation of adequate red blood cells.
5. Kernicterus is the destruction of brain cells by invasion of indirect bilirubin.
6. Periodic apnea: no bradycardia seen in the irregular breathing patterns, True apnea: irregular breathing patterns lasting more than 20 seconds with bradycardia.
7. Small plugs of meconium may be pushed farther into the lungs if infant is ventilated before the airway is cleared.
8. Newborn respiratory rate remains between 80 to 120 after first hour of birth, mild retractions, marked cyanosis, chest x-ray reveals fluid in central lung fields with adequate aeration; syndrome peaks in 3 hours and tends to fade by 2 hours.

PART 2

1. initiation and maintenance of respiration, establishment of extrauterine circulation, control of body temperature, intake of adequate nourishment, establishment of waste elimination, prevention of infection, establishment of an infant-parent relationship, development care that balances rest and stimulation for mental development
2. blindness; vasoconstriction.

SECTION THREE

1. B   2. C   3. D   4. D   5. D   6. C   7. B   8. A   9. C   10. C   11. A   12. A

Chapter 27

SECTION ONE
PART 1

1. c   2. e   3. f   4. a   5. b   6. d

PART 2

1. c, f
2. g
3. j
4. k
5. e, i
6. b, d, h

PART 3

1. Height; weight
2. Maturation
3. Growth
4. Development
5. Anticipatory guidance
6. Cognitive

SECTION TWO
PART 1

1. Oral: infant; 1 month to 1 year
2. Anal; toddler; 1 year to 3 years
3. Genital; preschooler; 3 years to 6 years
4. Latent; school-age; 5 years to 13 years
5. Genital; adolescent; 13 years to 18 years

PART 2

1. toddler (autonomy)
2. adolescent (identity)
3. school-age (industry)
4. infant (trust)
5. Preschooler (initiative)

PART 3

1. preschooler (reciprocity)
2. adolescent (postconventional)
3. infant (prereligious)
4. toddler (punishment-obedience)
5. young school-age (conventional)

SECTION THREE
PART 1

1. B   2. D   3. C   4. A   5. B   6. B   7. B   8. C   9. A   10. A

Chapter 28

SECTION ONE

1. B   2. F   3. D   4. E   5. E   6. C   7. G   8. B   9. A

SECTION TWO

1. provides parents with opportunity to ask questions; anticipatory guidance; observe for potential health problems
2. 2 months
3. 6 months
4. aspiration
5. 8 months
6. ventral suspension, prone, sitting, standing/walking
7. Check sources for lead paint, use protective caps for outlets; install gates at top and bottom of stairs.
8. learn different textures; provides the opportunity to kick and exercise and for parental touch
9. Gently wipe the teeth with cloth.
10. Change the diaper frequently, clean the area after each diaper change, and apply ointments and creams.
11. deficient fluid, too little bulk, tight anal sphincter, type of formula, high-protein diet, undiluted cow's milk
12. number of stools per day, color of stools, consistency of stools

SECTION THREE
PART 1

1. B   2. C   3. B   4. D   5. D   6. B   7. D   8. C   9. C
10. A   11. A   12. B   13. A   14. C   15. A

Chapter 29

SECTION ONE

1. b   2. d   3. a   4. c   5. f   6. e

SECTION TWO

15 months: walks alone, puts pellets into small bottles, scribbles voluntarily with a pencil or crayon, speaks four to six words

24 months: walks up stairs alone using both feet on same step at the same time, opens doors turning knobs, unscrews lids, speaks two-word sentences (noun/pronoun and verb).

30 months: can jump down from chairs, makes simple lines or strokes for crosses with a pencil, can speak full name, names one color, holds up finger to show age

SECTION THREE
PART 1

1. D   2. B   3. A   4. B   5. D   6. C

PART 2

1. I   2. A   3. A   4. A   5. I   6. I   7. I   8. I   9. A   10. A

Chapter 30

SECTION ONE

1. e   2. c   3. a   4. b   5. d

SECTION TWO
PART 1

1. large body build
2. slim body build
3. "knock-knee"
4. grinding the teeth at night

PART 2

1. Oedipus: preschool-age boys have strong emotional attachment for their mother. Electra: preschool-age girls have strong attachment for their fathers.
2. Preschoolers cannot comprehend that the same procedure can be performed in two different ways. Therefore, it is important to provide continuity when caring for this age group.
3. Seek to understand the child's fears. Monitor the child's exposure to environmental stimuli that may incite fears. Use a dim light in the bedroom at night.
4. Do not ask the child to recite or sing to strangers. Do not reward or punish the child in relationship to language fluency. Listen with patience. Do not discuss the child's difficulty in his or her presence.

SECTION THREE
PART 1

1. B   2. D   3. C   4. B   5. C

PART 2

1. I   2. A   3. I   4. I   5. A   6. A   7. A   8. I   9. A   10. A

Chapter 31

SECTION ONE

1. b   2. d   3. a   4. f   5. e   6. g   7. c

SECTION TWO
PART 1

1. clitoris; labia; penis; testes
2. 9

PART 2

1. Follicle stimulating hormone (FSH): stimulates growth and maturation of immature ovum in females; produces development of the seminiferous tubules and spermatogenesis in males. Luteinizing hormone (LH): causes the phenomenon of ovulation in females; stimulates Leydig cells in testes of males to produce androgens.
2. Gaining a sense of initiative is learning how to do things; doing them well is a step toward gaining a sense of industry. When a child's environment does not allow this sense of accomplishment, he develops a feeling of inferiority and becomes convinced that he cannot do many things that he in fact is able to do.

3. Decenter: ability to focus on other views besides one's own. Accommodation: ability to adapt thought processes to fit what is perceived. Conservation: ability to appreciate that a change in shape does not necessarily mean a change in size. Class inclusion: the concept that objects can belong to more than one classification (i.e., stones and shells may be gathered on the beach but they are different objects).

4. Be flexible when approving reading materials. Select readings that allow the child to complete a topic or finish in a short period of time.

5. School phobia is a child's resistance to attend school manifested by physical illnesses. The illness may be due to fear of separation from parents, fear of the younger siblings usurping the parents' love, overdependence, or overprotection by the parents. To resolve the problem, the entire family must be counseled. The parents must be consistent and firm with the child. Initiating attendance at school gradually, such as attending school for fewer hours, may prove beneficial.

PART 3

1. Teach child to swim; advise not to try to swim beyond capabilities.
2. Encourage use of seat belts; learn to cross streets safely; learn bicycle safety rules.
3. Wear appropriate gear; do not encourage the child to play beyond his or her capabilities.
4. Avoid unsafe areas; avoid strangers. Teach child to say "no" to and report persons who make him or her uncomfortable.
5. Teach safe use of firearms; keep firearms in locked cabinet with bullets separated from gun.

SECTION THREE
PART 1

1. D   2. A   3. D   4. A   5. B

Chapter 32

SECTION ONE

1. a   2. j   3. e   4. f   5. b   6. g   7. i   8. h   9. c   10. d

SECTION TWO
PART 1

1. mature; young
2. 3
3. decrease; increase
4. 13; 14; 15; 16; 17; 20
5. formal operations; 12; 13
6. sebum formation; comedones; bacterial proliferation
7. alcohol

PART 2

1. Private history-taking promotes independence and responsibility for self-care, and provides an opportunity for the youth to discuss matters he or she might not confide in front of a parent.
2. inadequate diet, poor sleep patterns, busy activity schedules (also emotional problems or boredom due to understimulation)
3. Intimacy: develop intimate (close) relationships with persons of the opposite and same sex; develop a sense of compassion for other persons. Emancipation: must overcome own and parental reluctance toward becoming an independent, responsible person. Values: determine who he or she is, and what kind of person he or she wants to be (must establish values of internal origin, not just mimic others).
4. Educating adolescents against cigarettes, smokeless tobacco, alcohol, drug abuse, and violence, and acting as support people for adolescents during times of crisis.
5. 13-year-old: impulsive; full of self-doubt; wants to be grown-up but still looks like a child; loud and boisterous; begins to long for the opposite sex and "falls in love" for the first

time. 14-year-old: quieter than at 13; more confident in self; searches for adult and older teen heroes to copy. 15-year-old: interested in approaching a member of the opposite sex; mainly physical attraction; "falls in love" frequently. 16-year-old: boys become sexually mature, though increase in height continues; both sexes are able to trust their bodies more; are more coordinated. 17-year-old: quieter and more thoughtful about interactions.

6. Any seven of the following would be correct: giving away prized possessions; organ donation questions; sudden, unexplained elevation of mood; accident proneness, carelessness, and death wishes; a statement such as "this is the last time you will see me"; decrease in verbal communication; withdrawal from peer activities or previously enjoyed events; previous suicide attempt; preference for art, music, and literature with themes of death; recent increase in personal conflicts with significant others; running away from home; inquiry about the hereafter; asking for information (supposedly for a friend) about suicide prevention and intervention; almost any sustained deviation (change) from the normal pattern of behavior.

SECTION THREE
PART 1

1. A   2. A   3. D   4. C   5. B   6. A   7. B   8. B   9. C   10. D

PART 2

1. A   2. A   3. I   4. I   5. I   6. A   7. A   8. I   9. A   10. A

Chapter 33

SECTION ONE

PART 1

1. C   2. D   3. A   4. B   5. D

PART 2

1. B   2. C   3. D   4. A

SECTION TWO
PART 1

1. air
2. geographic
3. school; inspiration; expiration

PART 2

1. introduction and explanation; chief concern; family profile; pregnancy history; history of past illnesses; day history; family illness history; review of systems
2. The height and weight fall below the third percentile on a standard growth chart.
3. cover test; Hirschburg test
4. Gently press the nostril closed and ask the child to inhale.
5. The tympanic membrane may be retracted; the malleus is extremely prominent; the cone of light is missing.
6. Perinatal infections; low birthweight; hyperbilirubinemia; bacterial meningitis; anatomic malformations

SECTION THREE
PART 1

1. C   2. B   3. A   4. C   5. D   6. A   7. B   8. B   9. A   10. C   11. A   12. A   13. A

Chapter 34

SECTION ONE
PART 1
1. g   2. b   3. h   4. d   5. c   6. e   7. a

PART 2
1. e   2. c   3. i   4. a   5. g   6. b   7. h   8. d   9. j   10. f

SECTION TWO
PART 1
1. Process recording
2. positive
3. environment; family members; family functioning
4. A. Psychomotor B. Cognitive C. Affective
5. Redemonstration
6. type; content; time
7. intermixed
8. memorizing
9. stages
10. interest
11. physical ability

PART 2
1. more economical; adds depth to learning; provides opportunity for shared experiences
2. assessing the child's current level of knowledge; the child's ability to learn new knowledge; the nurse's ability to teach the new knowledge
3. Visual aids help children see and better understand what will happen and how the procedure will affect the particular body parts.
4. Children learn to a point of saturation, at which point learning stops and does not continue until that information is absorbed and understood.
5. Nurses can help by consulting with schools and health care organizations to develop health teaching programs and by teaching such programs.

SECTION THREE
PART 1
1. C   2. C   3. A   4. D   5. B

PART 2
1. I   2. I   3. A   4. A   5. I   6. I   7. A

Chapter 35

SECTION ONE
PART 1
1. E   2. H   3. I   4. D   5. G   6. C   7. A   8. B

PART 2
1. T   2. F   3. F   4. F   5. F   6. T   7. F   8. F   9. F   10. T

SECTION TWO
PART 1
1. Play
2. perception; support people; coping experiences
3. (1) harm or injury; (2) separation; (3) unknown; (4) uncertain limits; (5) control
4. cognitive development; experiences; knowledge

5. observation
6. stress; stress
7. favorite toy
8. unknown; abandonment; mutilation
9. factual
10. Children may misinterpret nursing procedures as punishments and may be confused by terms used in explanations that often sound alike or have double meanings.

PART 2

1. infants
2. adolescents
3. toddlers
4. older children/school-age

SECTION THREE
PART 1

1. D   2. D   3. C   4. C   5. C

PART 2

1. A   2. I   3. I   4. A   5. A   6. A   7. A   8. I   9. I   10. A

Chapter 36

SECTION ONE

1. D   2. E   3. A   4. C   5. B

SECTION TWO
PART 1

1. Clean-catch
2. locating an appliance small enough, skin irritation
3. 15
4. nonadhesive

PART 2

1. Physical: upper extremity restraints should be used during intravenous therapy when the child has a scalp vein infusion in place, to prevent the child from touching it; a jacket restraint will help to prevent the child from turning, if necessary. Psychological: familiarize the child with the techniques and equipment that are part of the preoperative and postoperative care using an age-appropriate teaching plan. Physical: nothing by mouth for a designated period of time before surgery; washing the incision area; removal of barrettes, bobby pins, and dental appliances, if present; checking the mouth for loose teeth; dressing in hospital gown and underpants; checking for correct and legible identification band.
2. Any four of the following would be correct (see the text for detailed descriptions): side rails, clove-hitch, jackets, elbow, wheelchairs and carts, mummy.
3. Nurses can keep children free from disease so they receive a minimum of procedures. Nurses can provide health counseling regarding illness prevention.

SECTION THREE
PART 1

1. D   2. C   3. D   4. C   5. C   6. B

PART 2

1. A   2. I   3. A   4. A   5. A   6. I   7. I   8. A   9. I
10. I   11. I   12. A   13. A   14. A

Chapter 37

SECTION ONE
1. E   2. D   3. A   4. C   5. B

SECTION TWO
PART 1
1. Any four of the following: orally, intranasally, transdermally, topically, rectally, injectable, or inhalation.
2. weight, body surface
3. back
4. down, back
5. vastus lateralis muscle (anterior thigh)
6. Intravenous
7. heparin lock
8. immaturity

PART 2
1. The younger the child, the slower the rate of drug absorption, distribution, and excretion. Drugs are inactivated faster in young children than in adults but slower in newborns.
2. Upper extremity restraints should be used during intravenous therapy when the child has a scalp vein infusion in place, to prevent the child from touching it; a jacket restraint will help to prevent the child from turning, if necessary.
3. automatic flow infusion pump; fluid chamber; mini-dropper
4. Right medicine, right child, right dose, right time, right route, right patient instruction

SECTION THREE
PART 1
1. C   2. D   3. B   4. C   5. C   6. B

PART 2
1. A   2. I   3. A   4. I   5. A   6. A   7. A   8. I   9. A   10. I

Chapter 38

SECTION ONE

1. D   2. C   3. E   4. A   5. B

SECTION TWO
Part 1
1. conscious sedation
2. topical anesthetic
3. oral analgesia
4. visual analog
5. substitution of meaning

Part 2
1. Any two of the following are correct: a belief that infants and young children do not experience pain; a fear of addiction to pain-relief medications; a fear of causing respiratory depression.
2. Pain assessment in children might be difficult because some will suffer pain rather than report it because of fear, some will distract themselves by play, and some will sleep from exhaustion caused by pain.
3. The gate control theory holds that because pain travels between the site of injury and the brain where the impulse is registered as pain, gating mechanisms in the dorsal horn of the spinal cord, when activated, can halt a pain impulse at the level of the cord.

SECTION THREE
Part 1

1. A   2. B   3. C   4. B

Chapter 39

SECTION ONE

1. E   2. F   3. D   4. K   5. B   6. Q   7. L   8. C   9. I
10. H   11. J   12. G   13. A   14. P   15. R   16. N   17. O

SECTION TWO

1. Anencephaly
2. Arnold Chiari
3. meconium plug
4. Ortolani's click
5. subluxated hip; dislocated hip

SECTION THREE
PART 1

1. C   2. A   3. B   4. C   5. A   6. B   7. C   8. D

Chapter 40

SECTION ONE

1. D   2. C   3. H   4. A   5. B   6. E   7. F   8. G   9. K
10. J   11. I   12. L

SECTION TWO

1. medulla; pons
2. filter; warm; moisten/humidify
3. tachypnea
4. Any five of the following would be correct: anoxia, apnea, dyspnea, tachypnea, hypoxia, hypoxemia, hyperventilation, hypoventilation.
5. Po_2, 80 to 100 mm Hg; Pco_2, 35 to 45 mm Hg; O_2 saturation, 96 to 98 percent; pH, 7.35 to 7.45, HCO_3, 22 to 26 mEq.
6. first 24 hours, 5th, 7th
7. frequent swallowing, clearing the throat, increased restlessness
8. complete obstruction of the glottis
9. Any three of the following: severe inspiratory stridor, high fever, hoarseness, very sore throat.
10. beginning cigarette smoking, increasing activity, child health maintenance

SECTION THREE
PART 1

1. C   2. A   3. B   4. B   5. A   6. A   7. D   8. B   9. D   10. C   11. C   12. D

Chapter 41

SECTION ONE

1. E   2. D   3. G   4. B   5. C   6. O   7. F   8. M   9. N
10. I   11. J   12. K   13. L   14. A

SECTION TWO
PART 1

1. left; right
2. difficulty feeding
3. air; fluid
4. hyperacute, acute, chronic
5. A. tetralogy of Fallot B. transposition of the great arteries C. tricuspid atresia
6. tachycardia
7. Rheumatic fever
8. Any three of the following are correct: bilateral congestion of ocular conjunctiva, changes in peripheral extremities, rash, swollen cervical lymph nodes, changes of mucous membrane of the upper respiratory tract such as strawberry tongue.
9. Respiratory failure

PART 2

1. medication taken during pregnancy, nutritional adequacy, radiation exposure, vaginal or other infection, cyanosis present at birth
2. information about care, steps for follow-up care and emergencies
3. use of anesthesia to induce sleep, equipment used after surgery, cough and deep breathing exercises
4. The duration of innocent murmurs is shorter than with organic murmurs. Innocent murmurs are soft and musical; organic murmurs are harsh and blowing. Innocent murmurs are of soft intensity; organic murmurs are of loud intensity.

SECTION THREE
PART 1

1. C   2. B   3. B   4. C   5. A   6. B   7. A   8. B   9. C

PART 2

1. I   2. I   3. I   4. A   5. I   6. I   7. A

Chapter 42

SECTION ONE

1. C   2. I   3. F   4. J   5. B   6. H   7. D   8. A   9. E   10. G

SECTION TWO
PART 1

1. Autoimmunity
2. 6
3. A. hypogammaglobinemia B. Combined T- and B-cell deficiency
4. sexual; parental
5. gloves
6. allergen
7. reduce the child's exposure to the allergen; hyposensitize the child to produce a state of increased clinical tolerance to the allergen; modify the child's response to the allergen with a pharmacologic agent
8. food diary
9. ice

PART 2

1. Refer to Table 42-4; any two measures in each category would be accurate.
2. Seborrheic dermatitis has no itching, begins at birth to 6 months, rarely lasts longer than 1 year, and does not cause the child to become moody. Infantile eczema causes severe itching, has a usual onset at 2 to 6 months, lasts 2 to 3 years, and causes the child to be irritable and fussy.

3. Congential immunodeficiency disorders occur because the child is born with inadequate (or totally without) essential immune substances; secondary immunodeficiency disorders occur as a result of a loss of immunity due to factors such as infection (HIV), cancer, renal disease, malnutrition, immunosuppressive therapy, aging, or other stressors.
4. Skin testing serves to isolate the antigen/allergen to which the child is sensitive.

SECTION THREE
PART 1

1. C   2. A   3. D   4. B

PART 2

1. A   2. I   3. A   4. A

Chapter 43

SECTION ONE
PART 1

1. T   2. T   3. T   4. F   5. 5   6. T   7. F   8. T   9. F   10. T

PART 2

1. B   2. C   3. E   4. F   5. G   6. I   7. A   8. D   9. J   10. K

SECTION TWO
PART 1

1. Incubation
2. viruses, bacteria, rickettsia, helminth, and fungi
3. Rocky Mountain spotted fever
4. hookworm
5. Varicella
6. Warts
7. fatal
8. 14; 21; parotitis
9. orchitis

PART 2

1. Pr, M, Gl (if handling secretions), G (if infant drools)
2. Pr (if hygiene is poor), G (if soiling is likely), Gl (with bedpan)
3. Gl (touching infectious material), G (for direct care)
4. G (if soiling is likely), M (for close contact), Gl (when touching infectious material)
5. Pr, G, M, Gl

PART 3

1. The chain of infection must be intact, consisting of a reservoir, a portal of exit, a means of transmission, a portal of entry, and a susceptible host.
2. Circumstances that cause a child to be susceptible to infection include a lack of natural antibodies or immunization against infection, young age, gender, the virulence of invading organisms, poor body defenses (physical, chemical), and immune type.
3. The measles vaccine may cause tuberculosis to become systemic.
4. Any time the health care worker comes in contact with bodily fluids or blood, gloves should be worn. A gown, mask, and goggles should be worn if splattering of blood or body fluids is likely. Hands should always be washed before and after contact with clients. Sharp objects should be handled carefully. Refer to Table 42-4 in the text for reference to blood spills, specimens, and resuscitation.
5. Symptoms of scarlet fever are abrupt and include fever, sore throat, headache, rash, chills, increased pulse rate, and malaise.

SECTION THREE
PART 1

1. C   2. C   3. B

PART 2

1. I   2. I   3. A   4. I   5. I   6. A   7. I   8. A   9. I   10. A

Chapter 44

SECTION ONE

1. C   2. G   3. A   4. E   5. B   6. I   7. D   8. J   9. H   10. F

SECTION TWO
PART 1

1. Platelets/thrombocytes
2. Bone marrow transfusion
3. Hemolysis
4. Erythrocytes
5. Graft-versus-host disease (GVHD)

PART 2

1. Congenital anemia is inherited as an autosomal recessive trait. During childhood through adolescence the child may begin to experience a reduction of all blood cells. Acquired anemia is caused by environmental insults (e.g., lead poisoning) or the therapeutic use of drugs (e.g., chloramphenicol or chemotherapy drugs).
2. Long-term infusions of packed red cells increase circulating iron levels to toxicity, and chelation therapy is necessary.

SECTION THREE
PART 1

1. B   2. A   3. D   4. D   5. C

Chapter 45

SECTION ONE

1. C   2. B   3. G   4. A   5. D   6. E

SECTION TWO
PART 1

1. Any five of the following would be accurate: vomiting, elevated plasma pH >7.45, elevated plasma bicarbonate >25 mEq/L, elevated urine pH >7, normal or elevated CO_2 >40 mEq/L, base excess, confusion, slowed respiration, twitching or muscle tremors (due to loss of calcium and tetany), decreased plasma potassium <3.6 mEq/L.
2. Any three of the following would be accurate: when it occurred (timing), the forcefulness of the ejection, appearance and smell, duration, amount, degree of distress noted in child.
3. parotid; sublingual; submandibular
4. Any six of the following would be correct: rapid respirations, rapid thready pulse, weight loss, sunken eyes, depressed fontanelles, pale cool skin, poor skin turgor, dry mucous membranes, oliguria, irritability, lethargy, confusion.
5. Crying; drawing both legs up toward the chest; playingchapxc for short intervals then crying profusely; vomitus containing bile; elevated temperature; increased white blood cell count; rapid pulse if necrosis has occurred
6. Children have an immunologic response to the gluten factor of protein found in foods containing gluten (e.g., wheat, barley). When ingested, changes in the intestinal mucosa occur, preventing absorption of foods across the intestinal mucosa villi to the bloodstream.

PART 2

1. gastroesophageal reflux (due to neuromuscular disturbance)
2. effortless; nonprojectile
3. dehydration; alkalosis (Damage to the esophagus could also result.)
4. thicker

SECTION THREE
PART 1

1. C   2. A   3. B

Chapter 46

SECTION ONE

1. H   2. J   3. D   4. E   5. F   6. C   7. I   8. G   9. A   10. B

SECTION TWO
PART 1

1. creatinine
2. Vesicoureteral reflux
3. Polycystic
4. antigen-antibody
5. edema; hypoalbuminemia; hyperlipidemia; proteinuria
6. pale; oliguria; hematuria

PART 2

1. The urethra is closer to the vagina in girls, and shorter and closer to the anus than in boys, allowing organisms to travel faster to the bladder.
2. Primary enuresis occurs if bladder training was never achieved, possibly due to mental retardation. Secondary enuresis occurs as a result of physiologic problems such as small bladder, urinary tract infection, or allergy, or psychological problems such as a new baby in the family, high stress level, change in habits, or change in environment.
3. Nephrotic syndrome occurs insidiously with rare hematuria, marked hyperlipidemia, extreme edema, and mild hypertension, whereas glomerulonephritis occurs abruptly with profuse hematuria, mild hyperlipidemia, mild edema, and marked hypertension. The treatment for nephrotic syndrome involves a high-protein, low-sodium diet, whereas glomerulonephritis commonly involves a diet normal for the age of the child; however, protein supplement or restrictions may be individually required.
4. The acute form of renal insufficiency usually occurs from a sudden body insult, whereas the chronic form of renal failure results from extensive kidney disease.
5. Salt restriction needs to be individualized: some children need less sodium, some need no restriction, and some children need additional sodium.

SECTION THREE
PART 1

1. C   2. C   3. A   4. B   5. D

PART 2

1. I   2. I   3. A   4. A   5. I   6. A   7. I   8. A   9. I
10. I   11. A   12. I   13. A   14. I   15. A

Chapter 47

SECTION ONE

1. F   2. J   3. C   4. H   5. K   6. B   7. D   8. G   9. I   10. E

SECTION TWO
PART 1

1. varicocele
2. Gynecomastia
3. scrotum; rare (or painless); metastasizes
4. Mittelschmerz, abdomen
5. Balanoposthitis
6. Cryptorchidism

PART 2

1. External sexual organs in the child are so incompletely or abnormally formed that it is impossible to clearly determine the child's sex by simple observation; a male infant with hypospadias and cryptorchidism; a child with ovaries and testes; an oversized clitoris the size of a penis.
2. uterus; fallopian tubes; ovaries; ovarian support structures
3. Any three of the following are correct: drop in progesterone just before menses, vitamin B complex deficiency, endometrial toxin from ischemic tissue, hypoglycemia causing surge of adrenaline, low calcium levels, poor renal clearance with water retention.
4. Early child-bearing is recommended. Tubal scarring may have occurred during the disease process.

SECTION THREE
PART 1

1. C   2. D   3. A   4. C   5. B

Chapter 48

SECTION ONE

1. D   2. F   3. A   4. H   5. B   6. E   7. G   8. C

SECTION TWO
Part 1

1. insulin; glucose; hyperglycemia; ketoacidosis
2. 30
3. 2; 4
4. 1-2
5. 4; 12

Part 2

1. regulate and coordinate body systems
2. A. Oxytocin maintains labor contractions; antidiuretic hormone (ADH) conserves fluids; TSH stimulates thyroids; adrenocorticotropic hormone (ACTH) stimulates adrenal fluids; gonadotropic hormone is involved in the production of testosterone, spermatogenesis, and maturation of ovarian follicle; somatotropin is a growth hormone. B. Thyroxin and triiodothyronine govern the metabolic rate; thyrocalcitonin inhibits bone reabsorption. C. Cortisol regulates serum glucose and protein; aldosterone regulates sodium retention; androgens control male characteristics such as muscle and body hair growth; epinephrine and norepinephrine increase blood pressure. D. Parathyroid hormone regulates serum level of calcium. E. Insulin transports glucose and allows cell to use glucose.

SECTION THREE
Part 1

1. B   2. D   3. A   4. B   5. B   6. B

Chapter 49

SECTION ONE
1. D   2. C   3. E   4. A   5. B   6. G   7. H

SECTION TWO
1. central; peripheral
2. balance; coordination
3. A. cerebella B. motor C. sensory
4. cause; expand
5. disorientation/confusion
6. arterial
7. streptococcal
8. supportive care
9. preschool; 5; 5
10. A. tonic-clonic B. simple partial C. psychomotor D. absence

SECTION THREE
PART 1
1. A   2. A   3. D   4. D   5. A   6. D   7. B   8. D   9. D   10. D

PART 2
1. I   2. A   3. I   4. A   5. I   6. A   7. A   8. I   9. I   10. I

Chapter 50

SECTION ONE
PART 1
1. H   2. I   3. F   4. G   5. E   6. B   7. J   8. D   9. A   10. C

PART 2
1. T   2. T   3. F   4. T

SECTION TWO
1. Stereopsis
2. Orthoptics
3. Hyperopia
4. Coloboma

SECTION THREE
PART 1
1. B   2. A   3. C   4. B   5. D   6. C   7. A   8. A

Chapter 51

SECTION ONE
1. J   2. F   3. D   4. G   5. E   6. L   7. A   8. K   9. H   10. C

SECTION TWO
PART 1
1. epiphyseal plate; periosteum
2. 4
3. 1; 1.5; 20

4. thickening; enlargement; adolescent; preadolescent
5. adolescents; lift
6. 16; 3; 1; 3; 8; 12
7. rested; isometric

PART 2

1. The leg brace would cause the child, particularly an adolescent, to feel different from peers; the mobility limitations would also decrease opportunities for socialization with other children, resulting in isolation and decreased opportunity for development.
2. Encourage contact with school friends; arrange the bed to permit visualization of unit activities; arrange for visits from friends; maintain activity by involving the child in age-appropriate activities; tutoring may be needed.
3. Positive measures: massage the area under the cast with hand; apply lotion to the area; when possible blow cool air through the cast. Negative measures: avoid using coat hangers, knitting needles, or any sharp objects for scratching.
4. Walk on tiptoe for 5 to 10 minutes; practice picking up marbles with the toes; an older child could stand pigeon-toed and throw weight forward into the lateral aspect of the feet.
5. Functional scoliosis is caused by secondary physical or visual problems and is treated by correcting the underlying problem and encouraging good posture and spinal stretching exercises. Structural scoliosis is an idiopathic, often inherited, permanent spine curvature requiring long-term bracing or traction, or both. Slight curvatures may require no treatment except observation until age 18.
6. Milwaukee brace: a torso brace with one anterior and two posterior rods, leather pads, and a torso piece; used to improve spinal alignment. Halo traction: involves a metal ring attached to the skull with pins; used to stabilize cervical spine and reduce spinal curves. Bryant's traction: skin traction used for fractured femurs and for congenital developmental defects; used in children less than 2 years old. Buck's traction: skin traction used to immobilize fractured femurs in children older than 2 years old. Skeletal traction: the child's body serves as the counter-pull; used to reduce dislocation and immobilize fractures.

SECTION THREE
PART 1

1. B   2. A   3. C   4. C   5. C   6. B   7. B   8. C

PART 2

1. I   2. A   3. A   4. A   5. I   6. A   7. A   8. A   9. I   10. I

Chapter 52

SECTION ONE

1. B   2. J   3. G   4. C   5. A   6. H   7. K   8. E   9. F   10. D

SECTION TWO
PART 1

1. the injuring agent; the part of the body injured; the immediate care
2. eye opening; motor; verbal
3. Third
4. sterile
5. open
6. primary; safety precautions; children

PART 2

1. Provide written instructions regarding the child's care at home; provide a telephone number for the parent to call if questions arise; schedule a return appointment for follow-up care.
2. The body proportions of infants and children differ from the adult proportions on which the rule of nines was based.

3. These burns are often accompanied by respiratory tract problems related to airway trauma due to heat, carbon monoxide, and smoke inhalation.

4. Aseptic technique and appropriate barriers are necessary to reduce the risk of infection.

5. First-degree: Cleanse the area with an antiseptic; apply an analgesic and antibiotic ointment and a gauze bandage. Do not break blister, and debride broken blisters. Keep dressings dry. Second- or third-degree: Some measures include prophylactic antibiotics; daily debridement and whirlpool; overextend joints with splints; pain management with analgesics (see toddler nursing care plan). Electrical burns: Unplug the electric cord and control bleeding with pressure to site; monitor for airway obstruction. Facial or neck burns: administer 100% oxygen; monitor for respiratory distress; prepare for tracheotomy or intubation.

SECTION THREE
PART 1

1. C   2. B   3. C   4. D

PART 2

1. A   2. I   3. A   4. I   5. A   6. A   7. I   8. I   9. A

10. I   11. I   12. A   13. A   14. I   15. I

Chapter 53

SECTION ONE

1. C   2. D   3. F   4. G   5. A   6. I   7. B   8. J   9. H   10. E

SECTION TWO
PART 1

1. living; physical; chemical

2. nausea; vomiting

3. remission; sanctuary; maintenance

4. pallor; low-grade fever; lethargy

5. node biopsy; biopsy; liver

6. necessary; his life

7. Ewing's sarcoma

8. Retinoblastoma

9. Enucleation

10. compression; invasion

PART 2

1. Any five of the following would be accurate: alkylating agents interfere with DNA synthesis; antibiotics impair DNA synthesis and destroy malignant cells; antimetabolites interfere with cell function; plant alkaloids interfere with cell mitosis; nitrosurea compounds interfere with DNA synthesis; enzymes remove substances needed to grow; steroids inhibit mitosis in cells; immunotherapy stimulates the immune system to attempt destruction of foreign or malignant cells.

2. Malignant cells take more than their share of nutrients from normal cells; nausea and vomiting from chemotherapy make it difficult for the child to maintain an adequate oral intake; stomatitis causes difficulty eating; and gastrointestinal ulcers and changes in fatty acid metabolism may interfere with absorption of nutrients. Some medications may alter taste sensations, which will affect appetite.

3. Stage I or II: radiation to lymph nodes above the diaphragm; stage III: radiation to lymph nodes above the diaphragm, retroperitoneum, and groin, and maybe chemotherapy; stage IV: 6 months of chemotherapy.

SECTION THREE
PART 1

1. C   2. D   3. B   4. B   5. B   6. D   7. C   8. A

PART 2

1. A   2. I   3. I   4. I   5. I   6. A   7. A   8. A   9. A   10. I

Chapter 54

SECTION ONE
PART 1

1. C   2. A   3. E   4. D   5. B

PART 2

1. F   2. T   3. F   4. F

SECTION TWO

1. significantly subaverage general intellectual functioning; an intelligence quotient of 70 or below with concurrent deficits; adaptive functioning
2. crying, suddenly followed immediately by giggling or laughing
3. Graphesthesia: ability to recognize a shape that has been traced on the skin; Stereognosis: ability to recognize an object by touch; Choreiform: aimless movements of arms.
4. Pica

SECTION THREE
PART 1

1. C   2. A   3. B   4. C   5. D   6. B

Chapter 55

SECTION ONE
PART 1

1. D   2. E   3. A   4. G   5. H   6. C   7. I   8. B   9. J

SECTION TWO
PART 1

1. The nurse
2. special parent; different; special event
3. alcohol
4. repeat/support

PART 2

1. The family is a disrupted one (family members are reluctant to seek medical assistance for medical problems due to fear of discovery of the abuse).
2. Abusive behavior is often the only role modeling for parenting the child has been exposed to; abuse becomes a learned behavior.
3. The nurse may tend to blame the victim due to personal feelings that somehow the abuse was deserved or provoked by the victim.
4. Place the infant on an age-appropriate diet, and if the child gains weight the problem is probably nonorganic.
5. below the third percentile for standard weight and height; motor and social developmental delays; lethargy, poor muscle tone; reluctance to initiate human contact; few comfort-seeking behaviors

SECTION THREE
PART 1

1. B   2. D   3. A   4. D   5. D   6. C   7. D   8. D   9. A

PART 2

1. I   2. I   3. A   4. A   5. I   6. A   7. I   8. A   9. A   10. I

Chapter 56

SECTION ONE
PART 1

1. C   2. E   3. B   4. A   5. D

PART 2

1. I   2. D   3. E   4. G   5. J   6. H   7. A   8. C   9. F   10. B

SECTION TWO
PART 1

1. their perception of the event; the type and kind of support they receive from people around them; the ways that they have found successful in coping with stressful situations in the past
2. available transportation; financial situation/insurance coverage; language barriers; helpful health care providers
3. Any two of the following would be accurate: fear, feelings of failure, possibly all stages of grief
4. congenital anomalies; immunizations

PART 2

1. With a nondisabling chronic illness, the child and family feel they have some control over the course of the illness. The illness would likely have minimal effect on family functioning, although some adjustments may be needed. A disabling illness will likely have a great effect on a family due to many role changes, feelings of helplessness and powerlessness, and lack of control or ability to alter the course of the disease.
2. Youth may impair the ability of parents to care for a child due to lack of experience and problem-solving ability, making all phases of parenting more difficult than for older parents. However, youth may be an advantage to parents because young parents tend to be more flexible and creative in parenting than older parents.
3. Should the child's parents die, the disabled or chronically ill child will need a designated caretaker; the will would provide for this care, should it be needed.
4. Determining the effectiveness of the plan of care might help the nurse to better plan assistance for the next terminally ill child and family.
5. Any three of the following would be accurate: continue active conversation, use silence therapeutically, use the words "dying" and "death" when appropriate, preserve the dying child's defenses, sit with the child at night and allow the child to talk about dying if desired, be supportive, be aware that not all people's beliefs are the same as yours.

SECTION THREE
PART 1

1. C   2. C   3. C   4. C   5. B